Praise for
Ten Essentials to Save Your Vision

Dr. Edward Kondrot is a messenger of hope. He truly embodies the ideal of "First, do no harm." His careful explanations of the ten essentials to eye health serve as a powerful introduction and reinforcement to those who choose this road less traveled. I found this book fascinating. I am grateful beyond words to have this visionary doctor give me a huge measure of control over the gift of sight.

-Dianne Cecchett

Since relocating to the Phoenix area in the summer of 2006, I have consulted with and been treated by Dr. Kondrot for age-related macular degeneration and cataracts in both eyes. Both of these conditions are continually improving (as is my eyesight), both functionally and in acuity, as a result of following the lifestyle changes and therapies Dr. Kondrot espouses. This, his latest book, is a cornucopia of great information on eye health and the treatments available to reverse eye problems. As with most successful therapies, the patient needs to accept responsibility for needed lifestyle changes, which Dr. Kondrot has detailed in this book.

-Louis Drummond

Most doctors who treat eye disease and prescribe glasses mean well. However, their training is overwhelmingly biased toward the standard treatment of prescription glasses and surgery. They have no background in nutrition or non-conventional approaches to treating problems with the eyes. Most optometrists and ophthalmologists treat the eyes as isolated parts of the body. The connection between overall health and eye health is not even addressed during mainstream eye exams.

That is why this book, Ten Essentials to Save Your Vision, is so very valuable. I don't believe there is a better book in which to find so much information that is both current and thorough on the subject of alternative treatments for the eyes.

The wonderful benefit of the book is its extensive coverage of nutrition, vitamins, drinking water, toxicities in our environment, and exercise, etc. Not only will our eyes improve when we apply the information to our daily lives, but our overall health will also reap big rewards. We may be able to prevent other health problems because of the valuable information in the book.

Most people, if given the chance, want to take control of their own health. Dr. Kondrot has done the research for us and we now have choices to make.

This book needs to be in the hands of all doctors treating eye diseases. We need these treatment options available in our local communities.

Unfortunately, it is hard to find practitioners able to perform some of the recommended treatments. Some of *the therapies involve a cost. If more doctors were trained in using the treatments, the cost might be lower.*

The Bates Method and other therapies described in the book are not widely accepted in the medical community. We need more controlled studies so that the leaders of institutions training our doctors will recognize the benefits.

We need to educate ourselves—and our eye doctors! This very readable book is a good start. Get this eye-opening book into the hands of as many people as possible, especially those treating our eyes and those training our doctors. Continue studying and writing about the research being done here and in other countries.

-Joyce Hill

As a registered nurse, I have seen the long-term problems and side effects that go along with treating symptoms rather than the underlying causes of disease. This book is for anyone who wants to take control of his or her health and vision by addressing the processes that lead to macular degeneration, along with finding out what critical steps need to be taken to improve sight and to reverse AMD.

-Leslie Degner, RN, BSN
http://www.webrn-maculardegeneration.com/

Writing in a conversational, breezy, and easily understood style, Dr. Kondrot has packed this book with essential information and advice. This is an essential read for those who desire to maintain or improve their eye and vision health. He includes chapters on a variety of modalities readers can incorporate in their lives to improve their vision, from nutrition and supplements to microcurrent and stem cell therapy. Definitely a must-read!

-Margaret Smith

Ten Essentials to Save Your Vision discusses many factors that have a bearing on sight and functional vision. Not only does this book give information on how to regain sight after injury or disease, it also gives valuable information on how to stay healthy. It treats the person as a whole, not segmented in parts.

-Norman L. Elliott, OD

If you have eye problems, please don't surrender to allowing "normal disease progression" while your eye doctor watches. The suggestions in this book are clear, straightforward, logical, and, in my experience, effective. I can assure you that even if your health challenges are not in your eyes, the suggestions in this book will go very far to assisting your body in healing. Remember, whatever helps any cell in your body to recover will be of assistance to every other cell, since your body is an integrated whole.

I could go on and on about different healing modalities, but it's better now that you hear this from Dr. Kondrot. Enjoy your journey back to health!

-Dr. Robert Rowen
Editor of *Second Opinion* Newsletter

Thank you for the opportunity to review this exciting book. Dr. Kondrot's down-to-earth ability to explain even the most difficult concepts makes the book easy to read. Several items that caught my "eye" were zinc deficiency, postural deficiency syndrome, and how seven of twelve cranial nerves are related to the eyes. Dr. Kondrot says, "We all have a personal Grizzly Bear." Regardless of one's eye condition, Dr. Kondrot's primary concern is "to convince you [and me] to invest in [our] health. It is [our] most important asset."

-Rosalyn Fast, BEd

Dr. Kondrot has written a book that can be an integrative primer for just about any organ system in the body, including the eyes. It is a basic "Handbook for Healthy Living" as well as a very exacting and common sense therapy program for eye diseases. It should be required reading for all students in traditional medical schools, all students in American high school and colleges, and anyone who wants a guidebook on how to live a healthy and complete life. I wholeheartedly recommend that YOU read it.

-Dr. Bruce H. Shelton, MD,
MD(H), DiHom, FBIH
Homeopathic Family Physician
President, AHIMA

There is an admonition that goes like this: "Put your eyes back in your head!" That is exactly what Dr. Edward

Kondrot, a holistic ophthalmologist, does in his ground-breaking book, Ten Essentials to Save Your Vision. He not only puts the eyes in the head, he also puts the head on the body. He maintains that our overall state of health has a great deal to do with the state of our vision. Dr. Kondrot insists that no treatment for eye disease, whether conventional or alternative, will be effective without the minimum groundwork of good nutrition, a balanced nervous system, and proper hydration. Ten Essentials offers a way for anyone to step up a personal health program. The beginner can start to improve eyesight by switching to organic food and proper supplements. The more sophisticated health reader can investigate the power of oxygen therapies and detoxification.

Dr. Kondrot is dedicated to self-empowerment as well as to rekindling hope in even people with the most advanced cases of vision loss. If African Dance can replace eye drops for glaucoma and palming (placing the hands over closed eyes) can reverse visual loss, I say go for it. No insurance, surgery, or drugs required. In fact, no doctors are needed. However, if you do want guidance on your vision-healing journey, Ten Essentials tells you how to find eye professionals who are trained in these alternative methods.

Ten Essentials is a template for complete health maintenance, health restoration, and the prevention of disease in any part of the body. Reading it, you will learn about methods that have been used for decades but have been spurned by established medicine: these are approaches your doctor will probably never mention. At the same time, you know that these techniques have been thoroughly researched and are being used with great success by a medical doctor who used conventional methods for many years before designing his own innovative program for his patients. As he says on his weekly radio show, Dr. Kondrot's mission is "to help you overcome your vision loss." In Ten Essentials, along with his previous two books on natural eye care methods, Dr. Kondrot lays it all out in a user-friendly, non-jargony way.

-Gloria St. John

Dr. Kondrot has written a comprehensive book that everyone should read to better understand how to protect his or her vision. As an optometrist who has practiced for over thirty years, I have used light therapy, nutrition, Qi-gong, vision therapy, and microcurrent stimulation on patients: all of these work to improve vision and function. The eyes cannot be isolated from the rest of the body and must be considered a part of the whole person. Take Dr. Kondrot's teachings to heart and you will find you can maintain good vision throughout your life. Don't wait until you have a vision problem. If you have a vision problem already, get this book and follow its advice. It is a must-read.

-Charles M. Steinberg, OD, NQA
Gesell Institute Of Child Development

Dr. Kondrot, thank you for giving me your wisdom and experience, tempered by your critical thinking, in this book. You have put this wealth of information and resource material into a logical, responsible, and highly useful format. I am looking forward to the cookbook and am happy to know you love to fiddle in the kitchen, as well as to fiddle with your violin.

-Vance Wright

Everyone with eyes needs to read this book. It provides insight into the essentials of sight. Not only does it include information not available from local optometrists, but the size of the print also makes it easy to read. Read, study, take appropriate action, and celebrate continued clear vision, courtesy of Dr. Kondrot.

-Patricia J. Allen

10
Essentials
to Save
Your
SIGHT

10
Essentials
to Save
Your
SIGHT

Fish oils are harmful for your eyes.

A 10 second test can save your sight.

Sunglasses can actually harm your eyes.

A lotion can reverse years of damage to your eyes.

Edward C. Kondrot, MD
Foreword by Dr. Robert Rowen

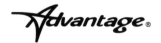

Published by Advantage, Charleston, South Carolina.
Member of Advantage Media Group.

ADVANTAGE is a registered trademark and the Advantage colophon is a trademark of Advantage Media Group, Inc.

Printed in the United States of America.

ISBN: 978-159932-329-9
LCCN: 2012941062

This publication is designed to provide accurate and authoritative information in regard to the subject matter covered. It is sold with the understanding that the publisher is not engaged in rendering legal, accounting, or other professional services. If legal advice or other expert assistance is required, the services of a competent professional person should be sought.

Advantage Media Group is proud to be a part of the Tree Neutral® program. Tree Neutral offsets the number of trees consumed in the production and printing of this book by taking proactive steps such as planting trees in direct proportion to the number of trees used to print books. To learn more about Tree Neutral, please visit **www.treeneutral.com**. To learn more about Advantage's commitment to being a responsible steward of the environment, please visit **www.advantagefamily.com/green**

Advantage Media Group is a leading publisher of business, motivation, and self-help authors. Do you have a manuscript or book idea that you would like to have considered for publication? Please visit **www.advantagefamily.com** or call **1.866.775.1696**

*This book is dedicated to my wonderful parents,
Edward and Lorraine Kondrot, who were always
there to guide and advise me.*

Acknowledgments

I want to thank many of the alternative doctors who have helped me over the years. These include Dr. Robert Rowen, Dr. Darren Starwynn, Dr. David Steinblock, Dr. Dennis Courtney, Dr. Dorothy Merritt, and Dr. David Nebbling. I would also like to thank the Arizona Naturopathic Doctors, especially Dr. Oddveig Myhre.

Special thanks to all the members of College Syntonics, especially Dr. Larry Wallace, Dr. Donald L. Barniske, Dr. Ray Gotlieb, and Dr. Jacob Liberman. These doctors all have shown me the healing power of light.

I would like to thank all the members of the Arizona Homeopathic and Integrative Medical Association, especially Dr. Bruce Shelton, Dr. Todd Rowe, and Dr. Abram Ber.

I am very grateful to the International Light Association for exposing me to the brilliant European Community of light energy healers.

Thanks to Ning Wu for developing the microcurrent technology that has helped so many people.

I thank the staff of KFNX talk radio for giving me the opportunity to broadcast the message of hope to so many people suffering with eye disease.

I extend thanks to Gloria St. John for her major contribution in editing this book. Her understanding of natural medicine contributed enormously to the final shape of this work.

My special thanks go to Advantage Media Group for putting the printed material into book form.

Special thanks to my Cousin Christine Kondrot for her very keen eye in helping to edit this book.

I would like to thank all of my patients for letting me be a partner in helping them improve their eyesight.

Lastly, my greatest appreciation goes to my wonderful wife, Ly, who supported me in this important project.

Foreword

by Dr. Robert Rowen

In today's "modern" medicine system, specialists have successfully dissected the human body into separate organs. There is a doctor for each one: kidney (nephrologist), heart (cardiologist), ear (otolaryngologist), bones (orthopedic surgeon), blood (hematologist), prostate (urologist), uterus (gynecologist), and so on. Let's not forget the eye (ophthalmologist). More often than not, medical doctors act as if each organ or system is separate and distinct from the others. And, worse, practitioners of modern medicine (which is more of a disease maintenance system than a health system) pay absolutely no attention to the fundamental causes of disease: malnutrition, toxins, and stress. Modern doctors act as if a patient's health problems are a natural deficiency of some petrochemical pharmaceutical. When it comes to diet, most doctors know nothing, and turn this most important of factors over to dieticians. Finally, and sadly, in my experience, most of these dieticians are totally in the dark about inherent biological nutrition but are terrific at calorie counting.

Once in a blue moon, an enlightened specialist sees clearly that the body works as an integrated whole, each organ and system supporting the others. Hence, it's possible that in such an integrated whole, a single problem, like macular degeneration, might have some outside underlying causes.

Perhaps you have a deficiency of magnesium, selenium, or zinc from eating low-quality food (as well as from eating crops grown in mineral-deficient soils). Perhaps you've accumulated a bit too much lead or other heavy metals, which have impregnated your sensory organs. Perhaps the problem is also related to other systems or to your body's entire health status! For example, vascular disease will affect the arteries that feed your eyes. In Eastern medicine, two organs—the liver and gallbladder—energetically control your eyes. Energetic dysfunction in these organs can cause eye deterioration. In addition, just maybe, you are deficient in an essential "nutrient" that comes from the sun: ultraviolet energy, which many eye doctors consider toxic to the eyes.

My own father was diagnosed with macular degeneration in 1990, when he was seventy-three. At the time, I lived in Alaska. My father periodically traveled from Florida to visit me in order to receive detox therapies (He underwent heavy metals chelation.) and circulation-promoting ozone therapy. He subscribed to my nutritional program, which is both oral and intravenous, and received hyperbaric oxygen therapy. None of these methods are conventional. They all support inherent healing processes in the body. For his own reasons, my father would not see local doctors; he only wanted treatment from me. Yet even with visits of several consecutive weeks at a time, which took place every other year, we kept my father driving until about 2005. At that point, he saw my friend and eye treatment mentor, Dr.

Kondrot, who assisted my father with frequency-specific microcurrent treatment. This immediately enabled my father to read at least two additional lines on the eye chart.

However, when one has a chronic degenerative condition, it's important to aggressively keep up with therapy. My dad did not. In addition, he developed other eye problems; his vision gradually deteriorated. Keeping him driving for fifteen years was still quite an accomplishment, especially since he had treatment at what I considered to be an intermittent rate (every two years).

Orthodox medicine has little to offer those with eye diseases like macular degeneration. That's because modern medicine can't look beyond a petrochemical pharmaceutical for treatment, or, in the case of eyes, a laser to burn and coagulate retinal tissue.

There are far better ways. Prevention is always first. Nutrition, detoxification, and stress reduction provide the means for your body to do what God designed it to do— protect and heal itself. Dr. Kondrot provides an outstanding template for prevention of disease and restoration of health, not just for your eyes but also for your whole body. Some of it may come as a real surprise, especially considering the eyes. For example, Dr. Kondrot bravely defies the conventional mantra that sun-related UV exposure is damaging in amounts we normally receive through daily life. In fact, he explains how UV deficiency might actually lead to retinal cell dysfunction.

Practitioners, including me, of ozone (oxidation) therapy, which is covered in this book, have seen some marvelous results from using oxidation therapy on eyes. I took an ozone machine to an Indian charity hospital and trained the doctors on its use. Months later, I was so pleased to learn that a child suffering from retinitis pigmentosa had had highly significant vision recovery from using ozone treatments.

Dr. Kondrot introduced me to a unique, 100-percent-safe form of healing. It involves delivering microcurrent therapy at specific frequencies. I witnessed what some would call miraculous, even instantaneous, results with this therapy in treatment of both eyes and other health/physical challenges. This is a form of therapy you really need to know about and is well covered in this book.

If you have eye problems, please don't surrender yourself to just allowing "normal disease progression" while your eye doctor watches. The suggestions in this book are clear, straight-forward, logical, and, in my experience, effective in many cases. I can assure you that following the suggestions in this book will go very far in assisting your body to heal, even if your health challenges are not in your eyes. Remember, whatever helps any cell in your body to recover will be of assistance to every other cell, since your body is an integrated whole.

I could go on and on about different healing modalities, but it's better now that you hear about them from Dr. Kondrot. Enjoy your journey back to health!

Ten Essentials To Save Your Sight

INTRODUCTION

by Edward Kondrot, MD, MD(H), CCH, DHt

Are you losing your eyesight? Are you one of the many people who are not satisfied with conventional eye care? Do you want to improve your vision? If you answered yes to any of these questions, I beg you to read this book so you can begin to restore your vision. Even if you follow just one step in this book, that can make a difference in your eyesight.

I am Dr. Edward Kondrot, a board-certified ophthalmologist who has practiced ophthalmology for over thirty-five years, as a traditional ophthalmologist for over 20 years and as homeopathic doctor who has worked with natural remedies for over fifteen years. I have written two bestselling books on alternative eye care, *Healing the Eye the Natural Way* and *Microcurrent Stimulation: Miracle Eye Cure*, and I host the weekly radio show *Healthy Vision Talk Radio*.

When I graduated from medical school with a degree in traditional ophthalmology, I felt that I had all the answers. I considered myself a very good surgeon and clinician, I knew all the basics of pharmaceutical drugs, and I was familiar with the latest eye treatments. However, there came a point in my career when I began to see patients whose vision was declining, even though I thought I had been helping them with surgery, drugs, and eye drops. They were also developing other health issues, which I feared might be related to these traditional treatments.

Personally, I passed a turning point in my understanding of traditional medicine when homeopathic treatment cured my life-threatening asthma. After this experience, I decided to devote my practice to alternative medicine. Since then, I have found these alternative techniques work in a very profound manner; in fact, over 90 percent of the patients I treat using these techniques experience vision improvement. My passion is really for alternative therapy, especially homeopathy: I believe these modalities can truly heal people, improving both their health and their vision.

The material in this book is derived from a series of lectures that I have been giving over the past ten years. I felt it was important to put all of the lecture material—and more—into this book.

Please do not waste any time—begin to learn the 10 Essentials to Save Your Eyesight now!

To your good health and clear vision!
Dr. Edward Kondrot

Nutrition and Supplements

I firmly believe that the greatest health issue facing us today is our diet. Unless we make some drastic changes to that diet, we can forget about saving our vision or expecting success when using other health-care modalities (I have discussed these modalities in my previous books, and will discuss several in the following chapters). Forget about microcurrent therapy, homeopathy, vision therapy, acupuncture, and the other techniques. Unless you have a good nutritional foundation, no other therapy is going to be effective.

BUY ORGANIC!

In my practice, my colleagues and I frequently talk about the 70/30 diet. The 70/30 diet is something we would like all our patients to begin using. This diet emphasizes 70 percent "organic" and living food, while the remaining 30 percent can be "non-organic" and cooked food. Why do we emphasize organic food? Simple. Every study that has been done comparing organic and non-organic food has shown an amazing difference between their nutritional values.

One study, done in the 1940s in the United States, analyzed the nutritional value of different fruits and vegetables' average serving sizes. Of course, at that time everything was organic by default. There was no systematic use of pesticides or preservatives. The study revealed that the average serving of spinach (about 100 grams) in the 1940s had about 158 milligrams of iron. Spinach today looks very good; all the leaves look perfect, nice, and clean. Yet today's serving of commercially-grown spinach has only 2.2 milligrams of iron in it. The iron content decreased from 158 to 2.2 milligrams. (Visit my website, www.healingtheeye. com, to discover links to other websites where you can learn more about the nutritional value of spinach and read about other related topics.)

In another study, conducted by Doctor's Data, a premier clinical laboratory with over thirty years' experience, researchers randomly selected different servings of organic food in supermarkets and then compared them to comparably sized servings of non-organic produce. In every one of the comparisons, the results showed that organic fruits and vegetables have five to ten times more beneficial vitamins and minerals than non-organic produce does. Not surprisingly, the harmful minerals (such as lead, mercury, and cadmium) were much higher in the non-organic food. The link to the Doctor's Data survey is provided on my website. For more information, you can also consult the following chart.

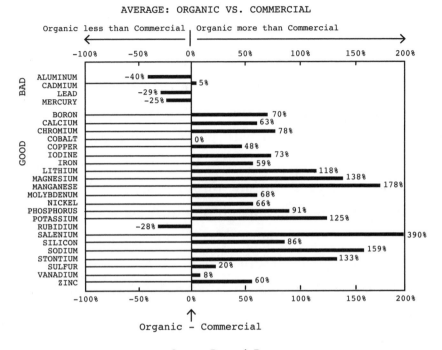

Source: Doctor's Data

While it is clear that all of us ought to consume organic foods (particularly produce), one of the biggest complaints I hear from patients is that they cannot afford to buy organic food. We are all cost-conscious; for some of us, this is due to living on a limited income, while for others, this is because we are in a recession. We are all looking at how we spend our money. However, I'll tell you that you really cannot afford not to buy organic food—not when you take the nutritional value into consideration. Even though you may be paying double the price for organic food, you are probably getting five to ten times the nutritional value.

Therefore, buying organic food is the first thing to do if you want to remain healthy. If you have a chronic disease or are suffering some type of physical ailment, the most basic thing you can do to improve your health is consume organic fruits and vegetables.

Another diet-related issue is the need for caution when purchasing imported produce; even if it is organic, it could still have been sprayed with pesticides and preservatives. Produce exposed to pesticides or other toxins can wind up on the market as organic through fraud, error, or environmental contamination, all of which are arguably more likely in the developing world. Of course, do not overlook the economical and health-related importance of supporting the growers in your area. When you buy from them, you are ensuring the continued availability of high-quality, local food.

These guidelines may help you begin to be more conscientious in your food shopping and preparation:

STEP 1

Read the stickers on fruits and vegetables. Many will tell you where the item was grown. If a sticker says "product of Mexico or China," choose a food grown somewhere else. If you are unsure about where a fruit or vegetable was grown, ask the produce staff at your supermarket.

STEP 2

Buy organic fruits and vegetables. Organic farmers in the United States are under strict regulations regarding their pesticide use. Choosing organic produce means that you are selecting food subjected to a minimum amount of chemical treatments. Some fruits and vegetables, known as the "dirty dozen," are more susceptible to the effects of pesticides. It is safer to choose organic versions of these items. See the list below to determine which foods are more susceptible to pesticides.

STEP 3

Shop at local farmers' markets. *Many small community farms grow fruits and vegetables without chemicals but they cannot afford to be certified as organic. Check out produce stands in your area and talk to farmers about how they treat their products. You may be surprised to find that fruits and vegetables grown closest to your home are the safest. In many areas of the country, you can join a co-op and have locally grown, in-season produce (that has not been treated with pesticides) delivered right to your home.*

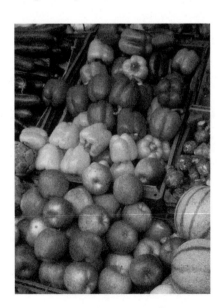

STEP 4

Wash your fruits and vegetables. *No matter where your produce comes from, wash it before eating, so as to clean off any pesticide residue that may still be on it. Use a mild soap and gently scrub the fruit or vegetable before cutting or peeling it.*

STEP 5

Dine in restaurants that have staff willing to tell you where they purchase the fruits and vegetables used in their dishes. *Many restaurants are moving toward using local produce, diminishing your chances of receiving foreign-grown items, but it never hurts to ask, just to be sure. This will safeguard your health and prevent illness.*

We have reproduced the list of the "cleanest" produce, or the items that normally have less pesticide residue, from www.thedailygreen.com:

Pineapple	Avocado
Asparagus	Sweet peas
Mango	Eggplant
Cantaloupe (domestic)	Kiwi
Cabbage	Watermelon
Sweet potatoes	Grapefruit
Mushrooms	

In contrast, here is the list of those items with the most chemical residue. These types of produce should always be purchased from an organic grower:

Apples   Celery
Strawberries   Peaches
Spinach   Imported grapes
Imported nectarines   Sweet bell peppers
Potatoes   Blueberries
Lettuce   Tomatoes
Kale and collard greens

With these differences in mind, it is critical that you seek out the local farmers' markets in your community. Get to know the growers in your area, or do what I do—grow your own food. I have my own organic garden in my backyard, so I know that what I am eating is organic, fresh, and of the highest nutritional value.

Prepare Food Right and Preserve Nutrients

Now, the other part of the improved-diet equation is to consume organic food in its most alive form. Once you start to steam, cook, or boil fruits and vegetables, you also start losing a great deal of the nutritional value. This holds true whether the produce is organic or not. Why? Because the protein has been denatured; cooking changes the food's chemical composition. A raw food diet is not only nutritious; it can also be lots of fun. Many people, when they hear the words "raw food diet," think of eating carrots and celery sticks all day or being hungry all the time. This does not give the full picture at all. It is amazing how creative you can be on a raw food diet. Recently, I made a raw, living meat loaf—with no meat in it. The meat loaf contained nuts, sprouted grains, tomatoes, and herbs. To create it, I combined the ingredients into a slurry mixture and then put the mixture into a dehydrator. After a couple of hours of dehydration, the mixture had the consistency of meatloaf.

According to Dr. Gabriel Cousens, author of *Rainbow Green Live-Food Cuisine* (2003), "Low-temperature food dehydration is a technique that warms and dries food that will not destroy enzymes." In contrast, Edward Howell points out in his book, *Food Enzymes for Health and Longevity*, that enzymes are destroyed when the food's temperature reaches 115 to 120 degrees Fahrenheit.

If you don't want to prepare raw foods, there are several you can purchase. Some companies even produce uncooked breads. Ezekiel 4:9® Bread, for example, is a raw bread made from dehydrated, sprouted grain and four beans. Typically, this bread contains wheat, spelt or rye, barley, millet, lentils, great northern beans, kidney beans, and pinto beans.

There are many fun and informative cookbooks and websites that feature raw and organic food, and that can be really helpful in introducing you to the whole concept of preparing and eating raw food. I have listed two great cookbooks in this chapter's resources section; the first one has the raw meatloaf recipe.

JUST SAY NO TO GMOS

Another important factor to consider when you are improving your diet and trying to become healthier is avoiding genetically modified food. This is another large health issue and a must for good health. In Europe, all genetically modified organisms (GMOs) are banned. However, here, in the United States, we are embracing the whole idea of genetically modified organisms. This trend originated with, and is perpetuated by, large corporations run by people who wish to profit from food. The Monsanto Company is one of the leaders of the genetically modified food movement. Recently, the federal government appointed one of Monsanto's former executives to take charge of food safety in the United States. I find this shocking; our watchdog agency is now a proponent of a highly dangerous food production method.

Although the press tells us that GMO food has more nutritional value and will solve the world hunger situation, this is not the whole truth—not at all. Every study that has been conducted on genetically modified food has shown this type of food has less nutritional value. Furthermore, these studies show that genetically modified food increases many types of health hazards, leading to more frequent instances of allergies, chronic diseases, cancer, and birth defects.

Dr. Arpad Pusztai, one of the first scientists to raise concerns about the safety of genetically modified (GM) foods, has conducted a landmark study on this subject. In the late 1990s, Pusztai, a respected molecular biologist, conducted research on GM potatoes for the Rowett Institute in Scotland. One of his projects was to study the effect of a Scotts Company product, Roundup®, on potatoes.

Roundup® spray is sold everywhere you turn. It kills every vegetative organism that it comes in contact with, making it one of the most popular weed-killers. Monsanto workers had come up with the idea to genetically modify plants so that Roundup® could be used freely to kill pests while not killing the plants. How did this come about, exactly? Observers noticed bacteria growing in the Roundup® waste dump. They decided to take that bacteria and genetically implant it into potatoes, producing genetically modified potatoes. Now you can spray Roundup® on these potatoes and it will kill everything except the potatoes. The company aggressively sold this GMO process to farmers, promising these farmers that they would be able to make more money, reduce labor costs, eliminate weeding, and gain a higher potato yield.

Doctor Pusztai decided to conduct an experiment to assess the nutritional value of Roundup® potatoes in comparison to other potatoes. He fed one group of rats the genetically modified potatoes, fed another group regular potatoes, and fed a third group regular potatoes along with actual bacteria from the Roundup® spray dump. Of the three different groups, only one consistently showed poor health results, such as stomach cancer, neurological problems, birth defects, allergies, and stomach lesions, as well as an overall failure to thrive. Can you guess which group that was? It was the group that ate the genetically modified potatoes.

Such GM practices are not limited to potatoes. Perhaps the most shocking statistic is that 90 percent of corn in the United States is genetically modified. About 80 percent of our soy products, and probably most of the cotton clothing products we wear, are genetically modified. These statistics are very, very frightening.

This food situation is, I believe, one of the reasons people are experiencing increases in chronic diseases, neurological problems, and eye disorders. We are eating genetically modified organisms in the United States despite research that clearly proves this practice is harmful. Many studies prove this. For readers such as you, who are interested in this problem, Jeffrey Smith has written a wonderful book called *Seeds of Deception*. Smith, a medical investigator, reports on the general issues of genetically modified food and what it is doing to our bodies and our health. The most frightening issue is that genetically modified food is an exponential problem. By this, I mean production and consumption of genetically modified food is increasing disproportionately in comparison to production and consumption of natural food. For example, one researcher stated that genetically modified salmon is taking over natural salmon; he predicted that we would not have any more natural salmon by the year 2012. Genetically modified corn is overtaking natural corn, too. If one farmer has genetically modified corn in his field, the pollen can blow over to the next (natural) field and cross-pollinate those crops. This type of cross-pollination helps explain why 90 percent of our corn is GMO.

The Problems with Corn

If we really look at the food products available in the United States, we start to realize that corn and its byproducts are in just about everything we eat. Cereal, for example, contains corn, while cornmeal is used as filler in many different foodstuffs. Another problem with corn is in one of its byproducts, High Fructose Corn Syrup or HFCS, has become the number one sweetener in the United States. There are three major problems with High Fructose Corn Syrup. First, High Fructose Corn Syrup is made from genetically modified corn. Second, during High Fructose Corn Syrup processing, mercury is introduced. I have read that there is more mercury in an average serving of High Fructose Corn Syrup than in the average can of tuna. Third, corn is metabolized in the body as a fat.

High Fructose Corn Syrup is used as a sweetener in all sodas, and consumption of these sodas is one of the reasons why more and more young children are becoming obese. This sweetener problem applies to several types of food as well as to sodas. I grew up in Pittsburgh, Pennsylvania, which is the home of Heinz ketchup. I love my Heinz ketchup. However, recently I looked more closely at the ingredients list on a bottle of Heinz ketchup. Guess what I saw on the label: "fortified with High Fructose Corn Syrup." High Fructose Corn Syrup is in everything.

You don't have to take my word for it when it comes to the dangers of High Fructose Corn Syrup. Take a look at this report from Princeton University describing an experiment in which one group of rats was fed a diet that included high fructose corn syrup, while another group was fed a diet that included table sugar:

Male rats given water sweetened with high-fructose corn syrup in addition to a standard diet of rat chow gained much more weight than male rats that received water sweetened with table sugar, or sucrose, in conjunction with the standard diet. The concentration of sugar in the sucrose solution was the same as is found in some commercial soft drinks, while the high-fructose corn syrup solution was half as concentrated as [that of] most sodas.

"These rats aren't just getting fat; they're demonstrating characteristics of obesity, including substantial increases in abdominal fat and circulating triglycerides," said Princeton graduate student Miriam Bocarsly. "In humans, these same characteristics are known risk factors for high blood pressure, coronary artery disease, cancer, and diabetes.

The problems with corn don't stop there. We've already talked about the dangers of corn, since most corn is GMO; we've also talked about the dangers of High Fructose Corn Syrup. Corn has a third problem. There is a mold endemic to all corn, even organic fresh corn from farmers' markets. This black mold is called *fumonisin*: it is a mycotoxin derived from *fusarium* and it is extremely neurotoxic. You cannot get rid of this black mold. The only way you can destroy it is by burning the corn.

I studied with Dr. Patricia Kane, a nutritionist who treats severe neurological problems through diet and specialized intravenous nutritional supplements. (Her website is www.patriciakane.net). I was interested in her aggressive nutritional approach to treating neurological disease. Because the eye is part of the neurological system, I speculated that Dr. Kane's approach would be very beneficial for treating eye disorders. I was surprised to find out that one of the first things she demands of all her patients is that they stop eating corn.

Now, if you are twenty or thirty years old and you have a healthy neurological system, corn is probably not going to hurt you. However, if you have a visual problem (such as macular degeneration or glaucoma) and/or a neurological problem, eating corn is going to contribute to that already full mix of toxins. Several studies conducted in Mexico have shown that a diet high in corn is linked to birth defects and neurological problems. However, all processed food has corn or corn byproducts in it, as you will discover once you start examining the ingredients in the food that you eat. This prevalence of corn and corn byproducts (and their associated neurotoxins) in mass-produced food could be one of the reasons why neurological problems are increasing for the general populace.

Although I am a real stickler when it comes to food shopping, I still make mistakes. Recently I bought a bottle of fruit juice: all-organic fruit juice. When I got the bottle home, I took a careful look at the label: it contained High Fructose Corn Syrup. Even though the juice had this ingredient, the company called it organic! High Fructose Corn Syrup is not organic. At that point I remembered my friend, Dr. Robert Rowen (he writes the *Second Opinion* newsletter www.SecondOpinionNewsletter.com), saying, "If it has a label on it, don't eat it." So, that's what I advise my patients to do too. If you go to supermarkets, shop only in the periphery, where all the healthy foods are. As you walk into the center of the supermarkets, the products' labels become longer and longer, including lists of preservatives.

YOU MUST BEGIN WITH DIETARY CLEAN-UP

A naturopathic doctor told me that when we are born, we arrive with an empty rain barrel (metaphorically speaking); as we live our lives, we accumulate more and more toxins in those barrels. When our rain barrels are filled with toxins and spill over, we get diseases. So, the number one thing we have got to do, in order to heal, is to stop putting toxins into our barrels—our bodies. For those of you who have eye problems, such as macular degeneration and glaucoma, or who have chronic conditions such as arthritis, your rain barrel is full. You've got to empty it, and you've got to prevent additional toxins from getting in.

Many of us live our lives participating in a subtle form of self-abuse. You go to McDonald's and eat garbage foods, and this diet does not seem to bother you. Then, all of a sudden, you reach a point in your life when you become really sensitive to food. You notice that if you eat a certain food you get upset or you get a headache. That's because your rain barrel is full. Those toxins have been accumulating in your body and now they are having an effect: you are "allergic." Then you read or hear about so-called miracle cures, where people offer testimonials such as this: "I began drinking berry juice and my arthritis and my vision got better." The reason why these types of cures work is because people are so toxic that any positive action they take, no matter what it is, is going to help in the short run. The problem with these miracle cures is then, all of a sudden, they do not work, and the patients need something else.

I am a firm believer in the idea that the first thing you've got to do in order to heal is work at your diet and become a stickler about what you eat, even though that is becoming more and more difficult. Obstacles include the continual increases in GMO foods and the difficulty, in some areas, of finding organic food. Learning to prepare and eat raw food also takes time and attention, but it has to be done in order for us to begin to rebuild our health properly.

Gluten Sensitivity

Another piece of the puzzle that makes improving food preparation and consumption even more complicated and difficult is that more people are developing gluten sensitivity. Gluten is hard to digest even for people who are not gluten sensitive; it is simply a very hard protein for the body to break down. In addition, it is even more prevalent than you would think. Gluten is even in licorice candy. How in the world did it end up in there? It is everywhere.

So, why are people experiencing an increase in sensitivity to something so prevalent? Believe it or not, one of the biggest reasons is due to eating bread containing wheat berries. Specifically, the problem comes from the way wheat berries are stored, which is in an environment in which they receive pesticides and preservatives. Wheat berries are stored for long periods of time, so despite the presence of pesticides and preservatives, mold still grows on the wheat. When we eat bread made from wheat berries that are moldy contaminated by pesticides, our body recognizes these pesticides and molds as foreign. In response to these foreign substances, we develop antibodies. At the same time, our bodies experience hyperactivity and begin to respond to gluten as a foreign material, too. At that point, we also develop gluten antibodies. This is the way food sensitivity—not just gluten sensitivity—happens for many people. You are living your life without any allergies at all; then, all of a sudden, you find you are allergic to a very prevalent food substance. Your body develops antibodies to such substances simply because they are delivered with preservatives and molds included.

I never thought I had a gluten allergy, even when I encountered some health problems. However, after I described some of my symptoms to Oddveig Myhre, a naturopathic doctor who worked at the Healing the Eye and Wellness Center, she advised me to follow a gluten-free diet. It is very difficult to go on a gluten-free diet, since gluten is so prevalent in our food: you've got to become a detective. However, after a couple of months on a gluten-free diet, I experienced many positive physiological changes.

In speaking with Dr. Myhre, I also learned she has observed a link between adrenal function and gluten sensitivity. The adrenal glands are small but very essential glands located above the kidneys on both sides of the body. They produce essential hormones that regulate blood sugar, help regulate the balance of salt and water and control the fight or flight response to stress. She says, "One of the things I do when I test my patients for adrenal issues is include a gluten sensitivity test. A couple of years ago, 10 percent of the people would [have] been gluten positive; lately, I have seen that at least 50 percent of the patients are gluten sensitive."

Remember, however, that gluten sensitivity is not the same as contracting celiac disease. In fact, scientists at the University of Maryland School of Medicine's Center for Celiac Research have proven that gluten sensitivity is different from celiac disease at the molecular level and in the response it elicits from the immune system. They have identified that 6 percent of the population (18 million people) is sensitive to gluten, and this percentage is increasing. If you want to regain your health, one thing you need to do is eliminate inflammation. However, if you have gluten sensitivity, eating products that contain gluten will create chronic inflammation in your body. This chronic inflammation, in turn, will prevent your body from healing. So, if you have a gluten allergy, you need to focus on gluten-free products.

Below are lists of foods containing gluten, particularly grains, as well as gluten-free foods, from the Mayo Clinic. In order to avoid eating gluten, avoid food and drinks containing:

Barley	Bulgur
Durum	Farina
Graham flour	Kamut
Matzo meal	Rye
Semolina	Spelt
Triticale	Wheat

Grains and starches allowed in a gluten-free diet include:

Amaranth

Arrowroot

Buckwheat

Corn (beware of GMO corn)

Cornmeal (beware of GMO cornmeal)

Gluten-free flours (made from rice, soy, corn, potatoes, and beans)

Hominy grits

Polenta

Quinoa

Rice

Tapioca

Even when following these lists, further vigilance is required. Check the product labels when buying amaranth, buckwheat, or quinoa. Each of these can be contaminated with gluten during processing.

One discovery I have made in treating patients is that even if all they do is cut out gluten, 90 percent of them will feel better. This is true even if they don't think they have gluten sensitivity. Sometimes other diagnoses are clues to gluten sensitivity. If your body has created anti-bodies to attack your thyroid, for example, and you have been diagnosed with Hashimoto's disease (this means your immune system is attacking your thyroid gland), you have a 93 percent chance of being gluten sensitive. In fact, I believe many other thyroid problems are actually due to gluten sensitivity.

So, to improve health, improving diet is absolutely crucial. I start my work with patients by coaching them to improve their diet first and foremost. We can't add supplements before improving the diet because supplements are just that—they are supposed to augment your diet, not replace it. If you want to regain your health, I cannot emphasize enough how critical diet is. Forget about doing anything else in terms of healing until you improve your diet substantially. It is unfortunate that most medical doctors don't really educate their patients about this important concept. They give permission for people to do anything they want in terms of lifestyle and dietary choices, and let pharmaceutical drugs address symptoms.

People need to recognize that going gluten-free is a major and a *permanent* lifestyle change; it is making a change to eating for your health and receiving nutrients from food. Food becomes your medicine. Some of my simple rules for consuming this medicine include the regulation of produce. If you are not diabetic, you need three times more vegetables than fruits; if you are diabetic you need five times more vegetables than fruits. Some patients think that fruits and vegetables are the same, and that they can consume ten fruits and one vegetable in order to meet their diet's produce requirement. No, it is the other way around.

MICROWAVE OVENS: DON'T KILL YOURSELF OR YOUR FOOD

After you've spent extra money to purchase the highest quality food, if you want to cook or heat some of it, do not use a microwave oven—for anything! Ninety percent of American households have a microwave. Microwaves are also present in dorms, offices, and break rooms in every workplace. Because of this, you may have become convinced that microwaves pose no harm to you, the environment, or your food. That is just what the microwave manufacturing industry wants you to believe.

Remember when microwave ovens first became popular, in the eighties? They came with some cautionary notes that most people soon learned and respected, such as "Don't stand too close"; "Check it for radiation leaks"; and "If you wear a pacemaker, don't go near one." Later on, a few more warnings were added: "Don't put any metal in the microwave"; "Watch out for cups of water boiling over"; and "Avoid microwaved popcorn."

Many of us began to think that if we just followed these simple precautions, we could use this most convenient and energy-efficient gift of modern life with impunity. Wrong,

wrong, wrong! At that point, people who said that microwaving food caused it to lose nutritional value were called fanatics. Other people might have said to themselves, "Well, maybe it does lose a little nutritional value, but the convenience of a quick heat-up is well worth it." The fact that many vegetables and healthy food can be purchased in easy-to-heat plastic packages adds to the misinformation surrounding microwaves.

I cannot really blame you for thinking that something the government has approved for use in homes, hospitals, workplaces, and schools must be safe. However, few of us consider the fact that the microwave, a common kitchen appliance, is actually a powerful machine capable of emitting up to 2,000 watts of electricity and heating food to over 200 degrees Fahrenheit. The real dangers of microwave cooking have been systematically suppressed. I am not going to spend energy in this book telling you how to have your microwave oven checked to see if it is leaking radiation or to put a chopstick in your teacup when you nuke it so that you don't burn yourself when you remove the cup. Instead, I am going to tell you to *get rid of your microwave*. If that is too difficult or radical, vow *never to use it again*. Never.

The real danger of microwave ovens is that they alter food's cellular makeup. This, in turn, alters your blood chemistry. The more often you use a microwave, the more significant and permanent the damage becomes. Not surprisingly, research that shows microwaves' real effects has been done in other countries. The Russians experimented with highly sophisticated equipment and discovered that a human did not even need to ingest the microwaved food for the substances to be harmful. They discovered that exposure to the energy field itself was sufficient enough to cause adverse side effects. These side effects were so severe that Soviet state law forbade the use of microwave apparatuses from 1976 to 1987.

Swedish investigator Hans Hertel has completed the most conclusive research on this subject. He studied the effects of microwaved nutrients on human beings' blood and physiology. This small but well-controlled study pointed the finger at the degenerative potential of microwave ovens and the food they produced. The conclusion was clear: microwave cooking changed the nutrients in food so that, when subjects ate it, their blood suffered resulting degenerative changes.

Hertel conducted this experiment on eight healthy individuals, all of whom ate a macrobiotic diet. (A macrobiotic diet is based on vegetables, grains, and small amounts of fruit and fish.) Researchers kept these people in one location for eight weeks, where the subjects consumed food and milk prepared in various ways. Researchers drew and analyzed the subjects' blood before and after each meal. Through the study, Hertel discovered significant changes in the blood of the volunteers who consumed foods cooked in the microwave. These changes included a decrease in all hemoglobin values and cholesterol values, especially in the HDL (good cholesterol) value and the LDL/HDL (bad cholesterol/good cholesterol) ratio. The blood work showed a short-term decrease in lymphocytes (white blood cells) following the intake of microwaved food, which did not occur after the intake of all the other variants of prepared food. Each of these indicators points away from robust health and toward degeneration.

THREE REASONS TO THROW OUT YOUR MICROWAVE OVEN FROM THE GLOBAL HEALING CENTER (WWW.GLOBALHEALINGCENTER.COM)

The following are conclusions about the dangers of micro-waves from Swiss, Russian, and German scientific clinical studies:

1. Continually eating food processed in a microwave causes long-term, permanent brain damage by "shorting out" electrical impulses in the brain (de-polarizing or de-magnetizing brain tissue).
2. The human body cannot metabolize (break down) the unknown byproducts found in microwaved food.
3. Male and female hormone production is shut down and/or altered by continual consumption of microwaved foods.

Unfortunately, you cannot afford to wait until the mainstream media communicates these dire findings to make a choice about abandoning your microwave. Make your own decision to stop using your microwave oven for anything that you will eventually put in your mouth now!

DIETARY SUPPLEMENTS

I want to begin this section on supplements by discussing the mineral zinc because it is so important to vision and eye health—and so many people are woefully deficient in zinc.

Why is zinc important? Zinc is essential for just about every enzymatic reaction in your body. If you are deficient in zinc, all the enzymatic and biochemical reactions in your body are not going to work up to capacity. We also know that zinc deficiency is related to macular degeneration, based on the latest national eye health study. So, if you don't have adequate levels of zinc, there is a good chance that this deficiency will contribute to your eye disease. In addition, adequate zinc levels are essential for microcurrent therapy to work properly. (See Chapter 8 for a full explanation of microcurrent therapy.)

Jerry Tennant, MD, a good friend of mine who is a researcher and developer of microcurrent devices, will not even treat patients if their zinc levels are deficient. I cannot afford to do that because then I would not be treating anybody! I would just be giving people advice about zinc. I do think that microcurrent therapy will not work as effectively for you if you are deficient in zinc; so, if you are embarking on microcurrent treatment and want to get the maximum benefits, it is important to raise your zinc levels. Our goal is to aggressively try to get your zinc levels—and all the other mineral levels—up while we are doing these treatments.

First, however, let's examine why so many people are zinc deficient. Because of present-day farming methods, more and more of us are becoming deficient in minerals. I grew up on a farm in Pennsylvania and every season we rotated our crops. We grew corn, oats, and wheat one year; then, the following year, we grew beans and legumes. That system of alternation put nutrients back into the soil. Today, by using pesticides and fertilizers, farmers are able to grow the same crops year after year. By doing so, they are not putting those trace minerals back into the soil. This is one of the reasons why our commercial food crops are so depleted in vitamins and minerals.

I estimate that 80 to 90 percent of my patients are deficient in zinc, even if they are taking it as a supplement. This is hard to believe; what's the reason for this? Earlier in the chapter, we discussed how mineral-deficient soil is, as illustrated by the study comparing the dramatic decrease in spinach's iron levels over the last seventy years. Another reason is that most people are supplementing with the wrong kind of zinc. Most common vitamins marketed as providing eye care now include zinc oxide, a form of zinc that absorbs poorly. This is what lifeguards put on their noses as sunblock! Instead, I recommend chelated forms of zinc, such as zinc picolinate.

In our office, we routinely use a simple, ten-second evaluation called the Zinc Tally Test to determine a patient's zinc levels. We place a few drops of a 1 percent zinc sulphate solution under the patient's tongue and evaluate the taste sensation. Typically, if your zinc levels are normal, you will immediately experience a very bitter taste that will increase over ten to fifteen seconds. If you do not taste anything, this indicates you are deficient in zinc. Do-it-yourself tests can be ordered on the Internet if you want to test yourself.

I have observed that over 80 percent of patients I test score as deficient in zinc, even if they are taking it as a supplement. They may be taking a poorly absorbable form of zinc, as discussed above, or they may have a diminished ability to absorb. Everyone over the age of 60 has a diminished ability to absorb nutrients. This is another reason why eating organic, raw foods is essential. These foods will provide you with the essential digestive enzymes to help absorb nutrition, as well as with the vitamins you need for your eye health.

IS CHROMIUM DEFICIENCY RELATED TO GLAUCOMA?

Many practitioners consider chromium deficiency related to diabetes. Richard Anderson, from the U.S. Department of Agriculture, offers this positive assessment of chromium supplementation: "Essentially, all the studies using chromium picolinate supplementation for impaired glucose intolerance and diabetes showed a positive effect."

Dr. Ben Lane, an alternative doctor, has studied fatigue syndrome, a type of eyestrain that develops after long periods of reading using improper reading glasses. He measured an elevation in intra-ocular pressure related to the number of hours of close work performed by the eyes. During reading, a muscle inside the eye called the ciliary muscle contracts, helping to bring the reading material into focus. Dr. Lane believes that proper reading glasses are essential to help relax the eyes, reduce strain, and prevent an increase in pressure. Lack of chromium may also be another factor that contributes to this fatigue syndrome. Chromium deficiency causes the ciliary muscle to reduce its utilization of glucose, and glucose utilization is necessary for the eye's optimal functioning during focusing work.

According to Dr. Jonathan V. Wright, the red blood cells of individuals with glaucoma had less than one-half the chromium levels of those belonging to normal, healthy patients.

Where do we obtain chromium? Foods high in chromium are the following: heavy cream, eggs, molasses, red wine and red grapes, and fat in red meat. If you have glaucoma, you should begin to incorporate more of these chromium rich foods in your diet and also consider taking a supplement of at least 200 micrograms of chromium. However, it's not enough to seek out chromium-rich foods.

You must also avoid vanadium-rich foods because another study showed that vanadium, which is a major inhibitor of chromium, causes an increase in intra-ocular pressure. Foods high in vanadium include red wine, fish, commercially fed poultry, kelp and seaweed, and chocolate.

Wait! Red wine is on both lists! How can this be? In red wine, the amount of chromium is much higher than the amount of vanadium, so the net effect is more chromium. All the red wine drinkers who are reading this book are safe.

If you have glaucoma, test your chromium levels.

Based on current research and many alternative doctors' opinions, all glaucoma patients should have their chromium levels tested. Fortunately, a chromium test is very simple; it is similar to the Zinc Talley Test described above. At this point in my practice, I now perform a chromium taste test on all of my glaucoma patients. I am shocked that most glaucoma vitamins do not contain chromium (and disturbed that very few glaucoma patients have had their chromium levels tested). In contrast, my optic nerve support formula not only has chromium; it also has digestive enzymes, probiotics, and betaine –three ingredients that help in the absorption of nutrients. The key ingredients in this formula help strengthen the optic nerve and lower intra-ocular pressure.

REDUCE MACULAR DEGENERATION WITH FOLIC ACID

You may also be able to reduce your risk of age-related macular degeneration—and, simultaneously, improve your vision—by taking an advanced metabolite of folic acid called L-methylfolate. At one of my three-day eye health programs in Houston, Texas, led along with Dr. Dorothy Merritt, I learned some important facts regarding methylfolate. Dr. Merritt is a big advocate of investigating a gene defect that decreases the ability to metabolize folic acid. This defect is also related to elevated homocysteine levels in the blood. Elevated homocysteine levels trigger abnormal changes in the cells that line blood vessels. These cells are much like the cement that keeps bricks together. When the cement and bricks (these cells) begin to weaken, the risk of bleeding and blockage greatly increases.

Many doctors are now measuring homocysteine levels to determine if patients are at risk for cardiovascular disease. Recent research has revealed that up to 60 percent of the United States' population may have a genetic defect that prevents them from getting this important nutrient into their brains. Taking folic acid in its methyl form allows these people to use this nutrient properly. If you've had an elevated homocysteine level in the past, you may want to take a test that checks your blood for polymorphorphism, or a gene defect that decreases your ability to metabolize folic acid. The test is called MTHFR (which stands for "methylenetetrahydrofolate reductase").

We tested all five of the patients who attended the three-day program in Houston and found, significantly, that all of them tested positive for this gene defect. These results suggest that all patients with macular degeneration should be tested for this defect or, to be on the safe side, begin to take supplemental methyl folate. Dr. Merritt has tested over 2,000 of her internal medicine patients: 90 percent of them have this gene mutation. She thinks this mutation is why so many of her patients have mood disorders, cardiovascular disease, and nerve pain, and she claims to be able to reverse 80 percent of these problems by treating the patients with high doses of various methylated B-vitamins and N-acetyl cysteine (NAC).

I came across the following article, "Plasma Homocysteine, Vitamin B12, and Folate Levels In Age-Related Macular Degeneration," by Dr. Gunhal Kamburoglu, which strongly supports Dr. Merritt's observation. In fact, I am in the process of changing my Macular Support Vitamin Formula to include the important ingredients of methyl folate and methyl B12.

Intravenous Nutritional Therapy

I feel that if we eat a good and healthy diet, we should not need to take supplemental vitamins and minerals. However, and unfortunately so, most of us have been on a pathetic diet for ten or twenty years—or longer—and we are severely deficient in most minerals and nutrients. That's why we have to make that shift toward changing our diet. In addition, we may need to give our bodies a boost at the same time. One way to do this is through intravenous vitamin therapy.

If you have a chronic eye problem, or suffer from some type of degenerative disease, we recommend that you consider what we call Myers' Cocktail. Myers' Cocktail is named after John Myers, a physician from Baltimore, Maryland, who treated patients with a form of intravenous nutrient cocktail therapy for over twenty-five years. The Cocktail, which is delivered intravenously, is a fortified vitamin mixture that contains magnesium, calcium, and vitamins B12, B6, B5, B complex, and C. In addition, in our office, we have modified Myers' Cocktail to make it more specific for the eye. We achieved this by adding taurine, an essential amino acid for retinal function, and zinc, an essential mineral lacked by many patients with eye problems (as described above). Changing your diet helps you address a mineral deficiency over a longer period of time; intravenous nutritional therapy can help you address this deficiency very quickly. Many medical doctors are now certified in holistic medicine and recognize the value of Myers' Cocktail. Naturopathic doctors can also administer these cocktails (depending on the licensing in the states where they practice). To find such doctors, check the following websites: www.holisticmedicine.org and www.naturopathic.org. You can also check the American College for the Advancement in Medicine's website, www.acam.org.

Folic Acid Intensive Therapy

You may also be able to reduce your risk of age-related macular degeneration and simultaneously improve your vision by taking a highly absorbable form of folic acid called L-methylfolate. Recent research has revealed that up to 60 percent of the United States' population may have a genetic defect preventing them from properly absorbing this important nutrient. Taking folic acid in its methyl form allows these people to use it properly.

Multiple Vitamin and Mineral Supplements

In addition to the specialized formulas and supplements I have already mentioned, you can supplement your diet with a good multiple-vitamin formula. What are the key components of such a formula? When I say "good," I mean a formula that is compounded and produced by a reputable company. You cannot go too far wrong if you shop in a health food store. Some of the staff are very well informed and may be able to help you make a good choice. The thing to avoid is purchasing vitamins at chain drugstores or supermarkets. Yes, these vitamins may have the same ingredients and amounts, but they are produced in a compounding process that may have cut a lot of corners. In such cases, you will not be able to digest and absorb the nutrients properly. Yes, the supplements at health food stores will be more expensive, just as organic food is more expensive than non-organic food. I am trying to convince you to invest in your health. It is your most important asset.

I recommend specific formulas and supplemental products, as well as eye drops, for all three major eye conditions (macular degeneration, glaucoma, and cataracts) on my website. I update these formulas as needed, based on evidence provided by new research. For now, you may want to take a look at the following link: www.HealingTheEye.com/Vitamin.html. Vitamin and nutritional research for the eye is rapidly changing; I strongly suggest you contact my office or your local alternative eye doctor for an update on the latest recommendations.

Before we review four of the most important vitamins (A, C, D, and E), I want to talk about dosage. There are generally three levels of dosage to keep in mind when developing or modifying your daily vitamin intake program. One of the levels of vitamin dosage is that which is necessary to prevent disease—the disease that forms when a person is deficient in a vitamin. For example, vitamin C deficiency leads to the disease known as scurvy, which is characterized by anemia, skin hemorrhages, and bleeding gums. While few adults receive diagnoses of full-blown scurvy in the United States, many adults bruise easily or have gum disease. These individuals might be deficient in vitamin C. Another disease, called rickets, is characterized by softening of the bones, and is due to vitamin D deficiency. We cannot help but wonder about the rise of osteopenia and osteoporosis in light of conventional medical recommendations, made during the last several decades, to avoid the sun and minimize vitamin D supplementation.

The next level of vitamin intake is called the RDA (recommended daily allowance). This is the amount, as determined by the Food and Drug Administration, that persons in various age groups need daily. Each vitamin's amount varies by age, gender, and special circumstances, such as pregnancy. New terms being used for this measurement are DRI (daily recommended intake) and RDI (reference daily intake). These measurements are used to calculate nutritional content in government-sponsored feeding projects. Overall, most people with an adequate diet meet these minimum requirements.

The third measure, and the one that is recognized and valued primarily in natural health circles, is the therapeutic use of supplements to overcome a deficiency or address a disease. For example, the dose of vitamin B in the Myers' Cocktail is therapeutic. Many people take high doses of vitamin C to prevent or minimize cold symptoms. Therapeutic doses are used for short time frames only and are prescribed based on the philosophy that vitamins can act like drugs, correcting an imbalance in the body.

Vitamin A

Your mother probably told you to eat carrots to take care of your eyes. She was right. Carrots, like many other orange-colored food items, contain large amounts of vitamin A. So do organ meats, butter, cheese, fish, and some types of meat. Of course, we now know that these dairy and animal products may not be good components for the best "eye health" diet, so we want to concentrate on getting our vitamin A from vegetables and fruit. The vegetables that contain the most vitamin A, in decreasing amounts per serving, are carrots, sweet potatoes, kale, turnip greens, winter squash, collard greens, Swiss chard, and red bell peppers. To gain the maximum benefit, you should eat carrots and red peppers when they are raw.

Vitamin A is a very complex substance. It exists in three forms. One of these, the retinal form, is specific to the health of the retina, so we are most concerned with that. We have known for a long time that vitamin A is important for healthy skin and connective tissue, but new research shows it also is involved in fundamental cellular processes that produce the body's energy. Here is what Dr. Rowen says about vitamin A in a recent issue of his newsletter, *Second Opinion* (www.SecondOpinionNewsletter.com):

> *Researchers recently discovered that vitamin A can significantly boost your energy. And it can fight cancer at the same time. In fact, the results of the study surprised these researchers. They didn't realize just how intimately involved this vitamin is in your ability to make energy. Natural vitamin A (not pro-vitamin A or beta carotene) has three forms. These are retinol, retinal, and retinoic acid. Retinal is essential for your retina . . . Retinoic acid is essential for skin and bone growth.*

Vitamin C

Unlike vitamin A, which is fat soluble, vitamin C is water-soluble. This means that excess amounts are excreted through urine rather than stored in fatty tissue. Nearly all mammals, except for humans, can produce their own vitamin C. Humans must consume this vitamin daily for optimum health.

The general public seems to think that vitamin C boosts immune system functionality and may protect against viral infections—and, perhaps, against other diseases. In my experience, I have noticed that increasing vitamin C intake to prevent or minimize a cold or flu episode seems to work for some people better than others. One thing that has been proven, however, is that vitamin C can play a role in cataract health. Decreased vitamin C levels in the eye's lens have been associated with increased cataract severity. In some studies, researchers have observed that a decreased risk of cataracts is associated with subjects' increased dietary vitamin C intake and increased blood levels of vitamin C.

These results are a bit too speculative to prompt me to declare that there is a definite relationship between vitamin C and cataract prevention. However, this vitamin is so essential to health and overall metabolic functioning that I highly recommend people get as much of it as possible through foods and supplementation. By looking at the chart below, you can see how easy it is to obtain several hundred milligrams of vitamin C from food daily, especially if you adopt the 70/30 diet that I recommend (described above). Remember that organic, non-GMO, fresh produce has even more nutrients than commercially-grown food.

Food Sources of Vitamin C	Serving	Vitamin C (mg)
Orange Juice	¾ cup (6 ounces)	62-93
Grapefruit Juice	¾ cup (6 ounces)	62-70
Orange	1 medium	70
Grapefruit	½ medium	38
Strawberries	1 cup, whole	85
Tomato	1 medium	16
Sweet Red Pepper	½ cup, raw and chopped	95
Broccoli	½ cup, cooked	51
Potato	1 medium, baked	17

Vitamin D

Vitamin D has been the stepchild of nutritional supplementation for decades. For a long time, people wrongly assumed that this vitamin was stored in fat and so large doses of it should be avoided. Of course, another bad idea—completely avoiding sunlight—has contributed to the astonishing vitamin D deficiency found throughout the population. Boy, were these people wrong! Scientists conducting new research have found that almost every person with cancer or other serious condition is woefully deficient in vitamin D. What's more, the role vitamin D plays in calcium absorption—and therefore in preventing osteoporosis—is phenomenal.

Research shows that the older we get, the more vitamin D we need each day. In a later chapter on light and its healing abilities, I discuss the benefits of getting sun exposure each day; this allows the body to produce its own vitamin D.

When sun exposure is not possible, due to infirmity or weather, then be sure to take a daily supplement. The best form of vitamin D to take is D3, and many D3 products are available in liquid form. Ideally, you should be tested in order to determine your particular need for vitamin D3 supplementation. Some people take large amounts, such as 2000 International Units (IU), and are still deficient in the circulating vitamin. Patients should, therefore, have their physicians test their serum 1.25-dihyroxy D3 levels to determine the proper level of supplementation required.

This testing is very important because vitamin D3 supplementation can raise calcium levels to an excessively high level in a small number of people. Many older people take upwards of 6000 IU of D3 per day, even up to 10,000 IU, if that dosage is indicated by their blood tests. Be prepared for the possibility of forcing the issue of the test with your doctor if he or she is not aware of the new research on this most essential vitamin.

Vitamin E

Vitamin E is a fat-soluble vitamin with antioxidant properties that exists in many forms, both natural and synthetic. Dosing and daily allowance recommendations for vitamin E may be found on food and supplement labels; they are often provided in IU. The natural forms (for example, d-gamma-tocopherol) are usually labeled with the letter "d," whereas synthetic forms (for example, dl-alpha-tocopherol) are labeled "dl."

Practitioners have proposed vitamin E for the prevention or treatment of numerous health conditions, because of its antioxidant properties. However, aside from treatment of the relatively rare vitamin E deficiency, there are no clearly proven medicinal uses of vitamin E supplementation beyond the recommended daily allowance. However, scientists are conducting ongoing research on this vitamin's possible effect on numerous diseases, particularly cancer and heart disease.

Scientists at the Linus Pauling Institute believe credible evidence exists to prove that taking a daily supplement (with a meal) of 200 IU (134 mg) of natural source d-alpha-tocopherol may help protect adults from chronic diseases, such as heart disease, strokes, neurodegenerative diseases, and some types of cancer. The amount of d-alpha-tocopherol required for such beneficial effects appears to be much greater than that which could be consumed through diet alone. This larger amount is considered safe even for older adults, assuming they are not taking blood thinning agents such as warfarin, heparin, or aspirin, and do not have a vitamin K deficiency.

Lutein and Zeaxanthin

Lutein and zeaxanthin are two pigments found both in the body and in nature: they are present in the macula (in the eye) and in vegetables. These pigments have been isolated and added to many products sold as vision formulas. Taking one of these supplemental vision formulas is a good step for anyone who has or wishes to prevent getting macular degeneration. However, taking a supplement is no substitute for expanding your diet to include the wonderful and tasty foods containing these pigments. The vegetables with the largest content of these pigments are kale, spinach, parsley, collard greens, (cooked) broccoli, green peas, pumpkin, and Brussels sprouts. One thing all of these foods have in common, with the exception of pumpkin, is that they lose their green color and turn yellow when they age. When these vegetables lose their color this indicates that a chemical reaction has taken place to reduce the potency of this essential nutrient. This is a tip-off to the presence of these vital pigments in any food and another reason to seek fresh raw organic fruits and vegetables.

Lutein is also in orange and yellow foods, including egg yolks. It is perfectly fine to combine green foods with foods of other colors; in fact, such combinations make for a more varied and tasty menu. If you wish to supplement your diet with lutein, I recommend consuming 20 mg daily. Look carefully at your supplement formulas, however, because many contain considerably less than this amount in their recommended daily doses. The following chart reveals the top foods that contain significant amounts of lutein (in milligrams per serving):

Kale (raw): 26.5 mg / 1 cup
Kale (cooked): 23.7 mg / 1 cup
Spinach (cooked): 20.4 mg / 1 cup
Collards (cooked): 14.6 mg / 1 cup
Turnip greens (cooked): 12.2 mg / 1 cup

DIGESTIVE SUPPORT

Over the years, I have come to realize that a good vitamin formula supplement, one that contains all the key ingredients, is still not enough for good eye health. Many patients face limiting factors in terms of their digestion and absorption capabilities. This is one reason I have added three additional types of ingredients to my macular degeneration vitamin formula: digestive enzymes, probiotics, and betaine. Digestive enzymes are enzymes that break down large, poorly-absorbed molecules into their smaller building blocks. This facilitates their absorption by the body. Digestive enzymes are found in raw uncooked fruits and vegetables (another factor contributing to the 70/30 diet). To aid digestion further, I use a proprietary powdered form of digestive enzymes in my formula.

The second type of ingredient I've added to my formula, to assist patients with nutrient absorption, is a probiotic blend. Probiotics are essential bacteria that reside in the intestine, helping it to assimilate and absorb food. They are beneficial because they improve intestinal microbial balance, thus improving digestion. The last item is betaine, which also aids digestion. During the digestion process, hydrochloric acid converts pepsinogen, a zymogen, to pepsin, an enzyme, in the stomach. Pepsin breaks down proteins into smaller, more easily absorbed substances. As people age, their hydrochloric acid secretion may be reduced, which can result in decreased levels of pepsin. Without proper pepsin levels, the body has a difficult time digesting food.

I use betaine hydrochloride as a supplemental source of hydrochloric acid. The stomach can use this, in turn, to produce pepsin.

THE DANGERS OF FISH OILS

Recently, at a monthly meeting of the Arizona Homeopathic and Integrative Medical Association (AHIMA), I heard a talk by Professor Brian Peskin. Prof. Peskin is a leading scientist specializing in EFAs (essential fatty acids) and their relationship to cancer and cardiovascular disease. His talk focused on the harmful effects of fish oils. Contrary to widespread, long-term popular belief, fish oils are causing harm to the cardiovascular system and are increasing the risk of cancer. After his talk I was in a state of shock: I could not sleep that night. I immediately called my friend Dr. Robert Rowen, editor of the *Second Opinion* newsletter (www.SecondOpinionNewsletter.com). To my surprise, I discovered he agrees with Professor Peskin's research completely. His comments on the subject follow:

I have been feverishly studying the materials on fish oil. I don't recommend them anymore except in unusual circumstances. The parent oils are safer, cleaner, and better received by the body. ["Parent oils" are vegetable oil sources of Omega 6.] Fish oil is not good for oxygen carriage across cell membranes. Many fish oil studies were not well done. They have flaws. One major flaw is that they are not controlling the effects of fish oil against parent oils. Fish oils might do some good for some people who are truly deficient in omega oils, but the deficiency is in the parent oil. Give them parent oils and they do as well or better than [they do with] fish oil.

Fish oil is being pushed in gram quantities that are far greater than the body can tolerate. This use makes it a drug. Parent oils are foods. Let the body make them into derivatives in its own wisdom.

Then, I asked Dr. Oddveig Myhre to comment on fish oils from a naturopathic practitioner's perspective:

Fish oils have been shown to be beneficial in many health conditions; however, there are issues with fish oils. One is the quality of the fish oil being taken. Many people are taking fish oils that are either rancid (usually sold cheap[ly] over the counter) or fish oils that contain heavy metals due to the poor purification process [used on them]. An additional problem seen with fish oils is poor absorption of this type of supplement. Any patient that has had [his or her] gallbladder removed, or has had gallbladder issues in the past, most likely will not absorb fish oils properly, which could cause irritation of blood vessels and other tissues. Furthermore, as we age, our ability to absorb essential oils decreases due to a reduction in lipase function. Lipase is an enzyme secreted by the pancreas that breaks down fat-soluble nutrients (lipids). All of this should be taken into account when [prescribing] supplementing [to] patients with fish oil.

There are two essential fatty acids: omega 6 and omega 3. They must come from food and, to work properly, they must be organically raised and processed to guarantee full physiological function. Most of the EFAs (essential fatty acids) taken as supplements are derivatives, and they are taken erroneously in high dosages. The body makes these derivatives on an as-needed basis in very small quantities. Most fish oil consists entirely of DHA (docosahexaenoic acid) and EFAs in super large dosages, and taking these products in high dosages will actually cause harm to the body, not benefit it!

In several well-done studies, fish oils have been found to be worthless in aiding atherosclerosis, and, in fact, might make it worse. I mention this because fish oils have gained quite a reputation as a nutrient needed for keeping hearts healthy. Because I know that many of my readers will be surprised by these new findings, I have listed a number of studies conducted on the effects fish oils at the end of the chapter. If you look over these articles, you will find that fish oil causes brain damage in adults and infants. You'll also see another disturbing finding: Fish oil can adversely affect your blood sugar.

Fish oil just does not work. Its promotion is another example of finance masquerading as science; in this case, such promotion has resulted in developing a market for the waste products of fish and contributing to medicine's long history of mistakes and erroneous dietary recommendations.

Instead of fish oils, what the body needs, according to Prof. Peskin, are parental essential oils or PEOs. What are PEOs? They are plant-based formulations of oils. Significantly, they are not derivatives; instead, they come from the parent oils of omega 6 and omega 3 that are organically raised and processed. Consuming these oils enables the body to make the derivatives that it needs. Examples of parent oils include high linolenic safflower oil, evening primrose oil, flaxseed oil, pumpkin seed oil, and coconut oil. Naturally, if you choose to consume these oils, you will want to purchase products that have oil sources that are as pure and organic as possible.

All this sounds good but what are the facts? One study that has convinced me, as well as Dr. Rowen and others, to stop using fish oil and switch to plant-based oils was the "Iowa Study: Investigating Oils with Respect to Arterial Flexibility: Significant Differences in Biological Age Compared to Physical Age" by Brian Peskin and David Sim, MD. This study used photoplethysmography (PTG) to measure the difference in arterial flexibility between subjects taking PEOs and those taking fish oils. Photoplethysmography is a non-invasive test that measures the flexibility of arteries. It is a superb diagnostic tool for measuring arterial hardening. This measurement then can be compared to that of a known population, providing a person's biological age based on the degree of hardening.

The study's participants were separated into two groups. The first group of patients never had received any type of fish oil. After their baseline PTG was measured, they were started on plant-based essential oils. The second group of patients had been consuming various brands of fish oil for the past six months. They were asked to stop using the fish oil and begin using the plant-based oils.

The conclusions were astonishing! In the first group, after 2.4 months, an astounding 73 percent had an average improvement of nine biological years in their arterial age. In the second group, after 3.5 months, 87 percent of the participants had reduced their biological arterial age by 11.1 percent (on average). This study indicates that the fish oil has no positive effects on, and may actually be harmful to, patients. (Neither this study nor the others referenced at the end of the book even consider the toxic doses of mercury found in many fish oils.)

What does this mean? This data indicates that PEOs might be more beneficial than fish oils. If you are taking high dosages of fish oil and your vision is declining, I strongly suggest you try plant-based essential fatty acids for a few months and check if this makes a difference. I have started a comparative study to consider whether there is a difference between ingesting PEOs and fish oils when treating macular degeneration and other eye disorders. If you are interested, please contact my office. We are now recommending a plant-based PEO supplement for our patients.

In order to regain and maintain your health, you may need to alter several other components of your lifestyle.

We will discuss these in the next chapters, but for now, congratulations on beginning to work on improving your nutrition, since good nutrition is the foundation of good health.

ARTICLES

Stacpoole, P., Alig, A., Ammon, L., and Crockett, E. "Dose-Response Effects of Dietary Marine Oil on Carbohydrate and Lipid Metabolism in Normal Subjects and Patients With Hypertriglyceridemia," *Metabolism*, Vol. 38, No 10 (October), 1989, pages 946-956:
The glycemic [blood sugar] control of [all of] the four insulin dependent diabetic patients worsened during the fish oil administration.

Quinn, J. et al. "Docosahexaenoic Acid Supplementation and Cognitive Decline in Alzheimer Disease: A Randomized Trial"*Journal of the American Medical Association*, November 3, 2010, Vol. 304, No. 17, pages 1903-1911:
Conclusion: Supplementation with DHA [marine based oils] compared with placebo [no marine based oils] did not slow the rate of cognitive and functional decline in patients with mild to moderate Alzheimer disease. [Note: Since the condition was "moderate," patients were still quite capable of improvement.

Fenton, J. et al. "Link Between Fish Oil And Increased Risk Of Colon Cancer In Mice," *Medical News Today (Colorectal cancer)*, Article URL: www.medicalnewstoday.com/articles/203683.php#post, October 7, 2010; and Woodworth, Hillary, L., et al., "Dietary Fish Oil Alters T Lymphocyte Cell Populations and Exacerbates Disease in a Mouse Model of Inflammatory Colitis," *Cancer Research*; 70(20); 7960–9; 0008-5472.CAN-10-1396; Published Online First August 26, 2010; doi:10.1158/0008-5472. CAN-10-1396.

Veirord, MB, et al. "Diet and Risk of Cutaneous Malignant Melanoma: A Prospective Study of 50,757 Norwegian Men and Women," *Int. J. Cancer:* 71,600-604 (1997): *A significant risk was found in women who used cod liver oil supplement. [W]e found a strong increased risk for the women using cod liver oil, a supplement rich in omega-3 fatty acids (EPA and DHA)." [There was approximately 3xs more incidence of melanoma (the most dangerous type of skin cancer) in the cod liver oil users.*

The International Society for the Study of Fatty Acids and Lipids (ISSFAL) 4th Congress, which met on June 4-9, 2000 in Tsukuba, Japan, and was reported in the article titled "Omega-3 Polyunsaturated Fatty Acids, Inflammation and Immunity," by Philip C. Calder, Institute of Human Nutrition, University of Southampton, Bassett Crescent End, Southampton, UK

...[S]tudies indicate that at the levels used, fish oil [omega-3 derivatives] decrease a wide range of immune cell responses (natural killer cell, cytotoxic T lymphocyte activities, lymphocyte proliferation and produc- tion of IL-2 and IFN-y (1,2))...

"Women With Type 1 Diabetes Receive No Heart Benefit From Omega-3," *Medical News Today (Diabetes)*, Article URL: http://www.medicalnewstoday.com/articles/193107. php, June 28, 2010:

Consuming higher amounts of omega-3 fatty acids [as found in fish oil] does not appear to lower heart disease risk for women with type 1 diabetes, according to a University of Pittsburgh Graduate School of Public Health study presented at the 70th Scientific Sessions of the American Diabetes Association.

Pot, GK, et al. "No effect of fish oil supplementation on serum inflammatory markers and their interrelation- ships: a randomized controlled trial in healthy, middle-aged individuals," *European Journal of Clinical Nutrition*, 2009 (62), 1353-1159:

In conclusion, this 12-week randomized, double-blind placebo-controlled intervention trial did not show that 1.5 g/day n-3 PUFA [fish oil] significantly affected the serum inflammatory response in healthy individuals, nor did patterns of inflammatory markers. Thus, a healthy middle-aged population may not benefit from fish oil as an anti-inflammatory agent.

CHAPTER ONE NOTES

Raw Food Cookbooks

I Am Grateful: Recipes and Lifestyle of Cafe Gratitude
by Terces Engelhart with Orchid

Raw: The Uncook Book: New Vegetarian Food for Life
by Juliano Brotman and Erika Lenkert

Raw Alkaline Cuisine by Salomon Montezinos
(www.evolvewithflavor.com)

Physicians

Dorothy Merritt, MD
Mainland Primary Care Physicians, LLC
6807 Emmett Lowrey Expy @103
Texas City, TX 77591
(409) 938-1770

Robert Rowen, MD
www.doctorrowen.com
Second Opinion Newsletter
www.secondopinionnewsletter.com

Websites

Nutritional value comparison of spinach:
www.awakeningpotentialsblog.com/awakening-potentials/
healthy-eating

Doctors' data study on organic food nutrient content:
www.rawfoodlife.com/Articles_Research/Organic_vs_
commercial_food/organic_vs_commercial_food.htm

Pesticide residue comparisons:
www.thedailygreen.com

Study on rats fed high-fructose corn syrup (Princeton University):
www.princeton.edu/main/news/archive/S26/91/22K07/

Dangers of microwave ovens:
www.globalhealingcenter.com/microwave-ovens-the-
proven-dangers.html

Dr. Kondrot's eye formulas:
www.healingtheeye.com/ZINC/Vitamin_protocols.html

Studies

GMO Potatoes Experiment

Ewen, Stanley W.B., and Pusztai, Arpad. "Effect of Diets Containing Genetically Modified Potatoes Express-ing *galanthus nivalis lectin* on Rat Small Intestine." *The Lancet* 354, no. 9187 (16 October 1999): 1353-1354.

Macular Degeneration and Folate Levels

Kamburoglu, G., Gumus, K., Kadayifcilar, S., and B. Eldem. "Plasma Homocysteine, Vitamin B12, and Folate Levels in Age-Related Macular Degeneration." Published by the Department of Ophthalmology, Hacettepe University Hospital,

Ankara, Turkey. Graefe's Archive for Clinical and Experimental Ophthalmology Volume 244, Number 5, 565-569, DOI: 10.1007/s00417-005-0108-2. This is a quotation from the study:

Summary: The purpose of this study was to investigate the association of age-related macular degeneration (AMD) with plasma homocysteine, vitamin B12, and folate levels. This study suggests an association between elevated plasma homocysteine and AMD, regardless of the subtype of the disease. Further controlled prospective studies are needed to investigate the possible role of homocysteine in AMD and the effect of vitamin B12 and folate supplementation in this process.

Fish Oil Studies

Burr, M.L., et al. "Lack of Benefit of Dietary Advice to Men with Angina: Results of a Controlled Trial." *European Journal of Clinical Nutrition* 57 (2003): 193-200.

Conclusion: Patients consuming three fish oil capsules daily had an adverse affect. Prof. Peskin's note: This group had more cardiovascular deaths.

Fenton, J., et al. "Link Between Fish Oil and Increased Risk of Colon Cancer in Mice." *Medical News Today* (October 7, 2010). http://www.medicalnewstoday.com/releases/203683.php#post

Lands, William E.M., et al. "Quantitative Effects of Dietary Polyunsaturated Fats on the Composition of Fatty Acids in Rat Tissue." Lipids 25 (1990): 505-551.

Conclusion: This study showed that overdosing on omega-3 from fish oil can be dangerous to your brain health at any age. Prof. Peskin's note: Both of these studies conclusively showed abnormalities in brain tissue resulting from administration of fish oil.

Pot, G.K., et al. "No Effects of Fish Oil Supplementation on Serum Inflammatory Markers and Their Interrelationships: A Randomized Controlled Trial in Healthy, Middle-Aged Individuals." *European Journal of Clinical Nutrition* 62 (2009): 1353-1350.

Conclusion: A healthy, middle-aged person may not benefit from using fish oil as an anti-inflammatory agent.

Quinn, J., et al. "Docosahexaenoic Acid Supplementation and Cognitive Decline in Alzheimer's Disease: A Randomized Trial." *Journal of the American Medical Association*, 304, no. 17 (Nov. 3, 2010): 1903-1911.

Conclusion: Supplementation with DHA (marine-based oils) compared to placebos (no marine-based oils) did not slow the rate of cognitive and functional decline in patients with mild to moderate Alzheimer's disease.

Sacks, Frank, et al. "Controlled Trial of Fish Oil for Regression of Human Coronary Atherosclerosis." *Journal of the American College of Cardiology* 25, no. 7 (June 1995): 1492-8.

Conclusion: Fish oil treatment of six grams a day does not promote a favorable change in the coronary arteries.

Stacpoole, P., et al. "Effects of Dietary Marine Oil on Carbohydrate and Lipid Metabolism in Normal Subjects and Patients with Hypertriglyceridemia." *Metabolism* 38, no. 10 (1989): 946-956.
Summary: In this study, all the diabetic patients' blood sugar control worsened during fish oil administration.

Veirord, M.B., et al, "Diet and Risk of Cutaneous Malignant Melanoma: A Prospective Study of 50,757 Norwegian Men and Women." *International Journal of Cancer* 71 (1997): 600-604.
Conclusion: Users of cod liver oil had an approximately threefold increase in melanoma.

Von Schacky, Clemens, et al. "The Effect of Dietary-3 Fatty Acids on Coronary Atherosclerosis: A Randomized, Double-Blind Study [and] Placebo-Controlled Trial." *Annals of Internal Medicine* 130 (1999): 554-562.
Conclusion: At the end of two years, both groups' clogged arteries had worsened.

Wainwright, P.E., et al. "The Effects of Dietary n-3/n-6 Ratio on Brain Development in the Mouse: A Dose Response Study with Long Chain n-3 Fatty Acids." *Lipids* 27, no. 2 (1992): 98-103.
Conclusion: This study showed that brain development is vulnerable to high dosages of omega-3 fatty acids in fish oils.

Woodworth, Hilary L., et al. "Dietary Fish Oil Alters T-lymphocyte Cell Populations and Exacerbates Disease in a Mouse Model of Inflammatory Colitis." *Cancer Research* 70, no. 20 (August 26, 2010): 7960-9.

"Women with Type 1 Diabetes Receive no Heart Benefit from Omega-3." *Medical News Today* (June 28, 2010): see www.medicalnewstoday.com/articles/193107.php.

Hydration and Detoxification

Now that you are eating the right food, you can start repairing your body. We want to return to the rain barrel analogy, in which the rain barrel is empty at birth and becomes full of toxins over time. One of the best ways to help empty that rain barrel is through detoxification. There are many ways to detoxify your body, but the best way is to drink plenty of water. At our practice, the Institute for Healing the Eye, we recommend that each day you drink one-half of your body weight in ounces of water. And that's ounces of water, not pounds of water. We get calls all the time from patients, saying, "Dr. Kondrot, I can't do it. I can't drink half my body weight; seventy pounds of water is too much. It is killing me." The recommendation is half the body weight in ounces of water. If you weigh 150 pounds, you should be drinking seventy-five ounces of water; that translates to a bit over nine cups of water per day. One way to be sure you drink this much is to fill a container each morning with the amount of water you want to drink that day and continue to drink until the container is empty. Keep it in the kitchen or at your desk, or divide the water into several smaller containers.

Why is it important to drink a lot of water? Our body is 60 to 80 percent water. When we are born, we are about 80 percent water, but when we die we are only about 40 or 50 percent water. Dehydration is a contributing factor to all chronic diseases. Dr. F. Batmanghelidj, a brilliant Persian physician, wrote a book on the subject called Your Body's Many Cries for Water; its subtitle specifies, "You are not sick, you are thirsty." Batmanghelidj believes most chronic diseases are related to dehydration. What happens to many men when they get older? They develop prostate problems and then they drink less water, because when they drink water they go to the bathroom too often. Women often get weak bladders later in life, and then they cut back on drinking water. Thus, slowly, we all get dehydrated.

DEHYDRATION AND EYE DISEASE

One of the earliest changes that we see in the eye, which is related to dehydration, is macular degeneration. This condition results from an accumulation of waste products, which doctors call "drusen," in the eye. A doctor may examine you and say, "Oh, I see some drusen." What does this mean? The appearance of drusen is the earliest change in the macular degeneration process, occurring before actual disease or visual impairment has even developed. This condition results from retinal cells becoming constipated, or being unable to eliminate metabolic waste products in that area. This inability is significant because the retina has an extremely high metabolic rate compared to the rates of other areas of the body. This retinal cell constipation is similar to what happens when your bowels are not moving, and you don't drink enough water. You are going to stay constipated. So, by drinking more water you help to eliminate some of the toxins from your body, a process that works on both types of constipation. It is absolutely essential to drink water to help detoxify your body. When you are adequately hydrated, your body can employ many mechanisms that help release toxins. These include the kidneys, perspiration, tears, and bowel movements. All of these processes release toxins. Remember, the worse your diet is, the more toxins you need to release.

How Contaminated is Water?

We have already discussed the difficulty of purchasing and preparing healthy food. Similarly, getting a good source of water is becoming more and more difficult and complex. We probably all know that we don't want to drink tap water regularly because tap water is becoming so polluted. It includes chlorination, fluoride, and pharmaceutical by-products that people dispose of through the water system. As an article in the March 8, 2009 issue of *USA Today* states, "A vast array of pharmaceuticals—including antibiotics, anticonvulsants, mood stabilizers, and sex hormones—

have been found in the drinking water supplies of at least 41 million Americans, an Associated Press investigation shows." Another article, this one from the April 19, 2009 issue of the paper, adds: "U.S. manufacturers, including major drug makers, have legally released at least 271 million pounds of pharmaceuticals into waterways that often provide drinking water—contamination the federal government has consistently overlooked, according to an Associated Press investigation" (http://www.usatoday.com/news/health/2008-03-09-water_N.htm).

The Green Pharmacy movement is working hard to make more people aware of this problem. The movement's workers are attempting to persuade hospitals, clinics, and even individuals to return unused drugs to sources where they can be disposed of properly, rather than by people's usual disposal practices, which include flushing drugs down the toilet or putting them into the garbage (which results in them being added to landfills). Yet the problem is increasing much faster than they can handle it.

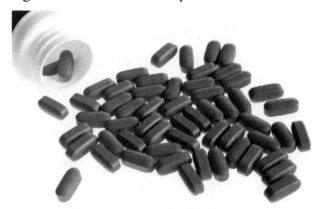

Do you want to drink these?

Here is some information on the subject from the CleanTechies' website:

Eighty percent of the U.S.'s streams and nearly a quarter of the nation's groundwater sampled by the United States Geological Survey (USGS) has been found to be contaminated with a variety of medications. This contamination is poised to worsen as the global appetite for medications swells. The drug industry sold $773 billion worth of drugs worldwide in 2008, more than double the amount sold in 2000, and, with an aging population and ever-cheaper manufacturing, pharmaceutical production is expected to grow 4 to 7 percent annually until at least 2013. Americans bring home more than 10 prescription drugs per capita per year, consuming an estimated 17 grams of antibiotics alone—more than three times the per capita rate of consumption in European countries such as Germany.

Hundreds of active pharmaceutical ingredients are used in a variety of manufacturing processes, in addition to making drugs. For example, lithium is used to make ceramics and treat bipolar disorder; nitroglycerin, a heart drug, is also used in explosives; and copper shows up in a variety of products, from pipes to contraceptives.

The Environmental Working Group (www.ewg.org) is also sounding an alarm on this topic:

[Our] studies show that tap water across the U.S. is contaminated with many industrial chemicals, and now we know that millions of Americans are also drinking

low-level mixtures of pharmaceuticals with every glass of water," said Jane Houlihan, EWG Vice President for Research. "The health effect of this cocktail of chemicals and drugs hasn't been studied, but we are concerned about risks for infants and others who are vulnerable. Once again, the press is doing the EPA's work when it comes to informing the public about contaminated tap water.

An Associated Press investigation published March 10th, 2008, found that the drinking water of millions of Americans may be contaminated by a wide range of pharmaceuticals. Most communities that have looked have found low levels of prescription drugs in their water—including cattle antibiotics, estrogens and other hormones —and the antidepressants that doctors are no longer permitted to prescribe to adolescents.

They miss some of the big issues. Our research shows mixtures are so prevalent," said Dana Kolpin, a U.S. Geological Survey water expert who launched a plethora of research in 2002 after finding pharmaceuticals in most samples taken from 139 streams in 30 states. "If there are any cumulative or additive issues, you can't just dismiss things so quickly."

On average, tap water in this country contains traces of antibiotics and other drugs (including hormones and even Viagra).

Where is the Pure Water?

For a long time, everybody believed that bottled water was good, even superior, to tap water. However, the situation is more complicated than that. The truth is, bottled water does not need to meet higher standards than tap water does; as a result, it may be more toxic than tap water, depending upon where you live and what your water source is. Drinking water from plastic bottles leads to other health issues, too. Studies have shown the plastic's phthalates and off-gassing are extremely harmful and contribute to many diseases, including breast cancer in women and hormonal problems in men.

Cancer survivor Sheryl Crow has a stern message for her fans about water quality: "Don't drink water from plastic bottles left in your car." Shortly after being diagnosed with breast cancer, Crow met with a nutritionist, and she was stunned when he alerted her to all the poor food choices that might have accelerated her disease. Now, Crow is keen to pass on advice to fans who want to avoid cancer at all costs—and her top tip is for people to be careful about their water containers. She explains, "If it [a plastic bottle] gets hot, it's omitting [carcinogenic] byproducts. To heat food in plastic, [or] to freeze food in plastic [can expose you to] carcinogenics, and cooking in olive oil at a high heat [is also dangerous]. If it's burning, it's carcinogenic. There are things we need to know and we [also] need to educate people about eating organically."

So what are you going to do? Where are you going to find your water? It's tough. Those of you who live in the countryside and use a natural well or spring water may have a very good water source. Yet those sources are becoming almost impossible to find. So, I recommend you invest in a reverse osmosis water-filtering unit. This is a simple device that goes underneath your sink and filters your water: specifically, the unit forces the water to pass through a filter that is too small to allow larger pollutant molecules to pass through it too. This results in water that is similar to distilled water. Your other option is to buy distilled water, but that can create more obstacles. Then, somehow, you need to find a way to transport the water in glass containers. I believe using a reverse osmosis unit is one way to guarantee that you have a pure water source.

The following description of reverse osmosis comes from one of the best sources for information on any type of water purification system, www.purewaterproducts.com:

Reverse osmosis is an advanced water purification method that was initially developed by the U.S. Navy to produce drinking water from sea water for submarine crews. It is a membrane filtration technology that works by forcing water under pressure through the very tiny pores of a semi-permeable membrane. Modern reverse osmosis units for the home combine membrane technology with carbon and mechanical filtration to produce highly purified, great-tasting water. In home units, water, driven by normal city water pressure, flows first through a carbon pre-filter, which removes organic contaminants including chlorine and its by-products. Next, it enters the reverse osmosis membrane, a very tight, sheet-like filter that allows water to pass but rejects dissolved solids like sodium and impurities like lead and arsenic. The purified water is stored in a small storage tank until it is needed. When the ledge faucet mounted on the sink is opened, the purified water is forced by air pressure through another carbon filter, which gives it a final polish and from there to the ledge faucet.

Now, the question patients always ask me is whether reverse osmosis water has all the minerals removed. The answer is, "Yes, reverse osmosis removes all the minerals." I recommend that you put a pinch of Himalayan salt (or a pinch of kelp) in the water, using a pinch per quart of water. This will replace many of the trace minerals. (In addition, remember that a diet including 70 percent organic, living produce provides more nutrient-rich food. This food is grown in better soil, which contains a lot more trace minerals.) What we recommend is that you use a specific type of salt, not just any type of salt. We recommend Himalayan sea salt, or a salt manufactured from an inland source, because the ocean is being contaminated. If you use regular sea salt, you will have higher traces of mercury, cadmium, and pharmaceuticals mixed in. Another option for getting trace minerals is to put a pinch of kelp (dried seaweed), into your water each day, but there is a risk of the kelp being contaminated, because it can be drawn from a polluted sea.

And what is Himalayan sea salt like? Here is a description of Himalayan sea salt from www.himalasalt.com:

Himalayan Salt is considered to be the most pure form of whole salt on the planet. Having never been exposed to impurities, and protected deep within the Himalayans for millions and millions of years, it was formed from the primordial ocean during a time of great tectonic pressure. This is important today, as even the highest quality sea salts come from current ocean waters that can contain heavy metals and harmful pollutants, and differ greatly from Himalayan Salt, [which is] also known as pink salt, Himalayan pink salt, Himalayan rock salt, Himalayan sea salt, [and] Himalayan crystal salt.

Another way to get adequate trace minerals is by ensuring they are in your produce. One of my patients, an agriculture professor, offered a suggestion. He said that one of the best ways to fortify your compost pile with trace minerals is to add items such as crab legs and lobster shells. Take them home from a restaurant and put them in your compost pile. Doing so will eventually enrich your garden plants. Ocean shells can contribute many of the trace minerals that may be missing from your soil.

COMPOSTING: THE COMPLETE CIRCLE

"What is composting?" you may ask. There are some simple instructions, as well as products, available at various lawn and garden stores or on Internet sites. The gist of composting is that it's a process in which you turn your kitchen and landscaping scraps (vegetable-based only—no animal products except eggshells) into rich dirt that can be added to your garden. Composting is highly ecological; it helps you reduce the amount of garbage you generate and, in fact, it turns that garbage into what gardeners call "black gold," or extremely rich soil. To succeed in composting, you will need organic material, moisture, airflow, and some insulation or container/containment area. As described on www.compostinstructions.com,

> *The perfect compost pile is damp without being wet, like a squeezed[-]out sponge. It should also be well aerated, with plenty of the oxygen that aerobic bacteria need. And it should have a mix of different types of materials. If you have just one thing, like grass clippings alone, or leaves alone, then it takes a really long time to break down. But if you have several materials and mix them all together, then they break down much more quickly.*

While there is an art to and some science involved in composting, it is a very forgiving endeavor. Pile too dry? Add water. Is it too wet? Wait; it will dry out. Many gardeners have been successful in composting by using leftover bins or containers that they already have. You can also invest in special systems that protect your compost from predatory animals while ensuring the best conditions for it to thrive. However, if you choose to compost, the important thing is that you just begin.

LIFESTYLE CHANGES EQUAL
GOOD MEDICINE

If you have a chronic disease, are losing your vision due to macular degeneration or another eye disease, or have some other physical problem, you need to take these basics of diet and hydration described in this book into your life—forever. You can't just depend on your doctor to give you a pill, some type of treatment, acupuncture, or even another form of natural therapy to cure you. Using these approaches, you will probably feel better for a short period of time. Afterwards, however, when you go home, eat your bad diet, and drink your polluted water, you will soon notice that you are not really getting better, and you will wonder why.

Consuming pure water is essential for those of you who are undergoing microcurrent treatment or any type of therapy to help detoxify your body. To help remove the toxins, you need that extra water, and it must be pure water. When we offer microcurrent treatment, we are simulating the cells, and those cells release more toxins as a result. Because you are releasing toxins, if you do not drink enough water, you are going to get sick; you will get flu symptoms, and your body will get achy. You can prevent this by drinking the recommended amount of pure water daily—not just during treatment, however, but for the rest of your life. The next section explains techniques that will help you get rid of toxins accumulated in your tissues, even if the accumulation happened long ago.

Heavy Metal Toxicity

As discussed earlier, most of the patients we see are terribly deficient in zinc, which is needed for vision, hearing, muscle function, and immune health. This does not mean that they are not taking enough zinc, though. Many patients have heavy metal toxicity. These heavy metals interact in their bodies in ways that are very detrimental to overall health. If there is a significant amount of lead present in the body, it will often replace zinc in the tissues.

Heavy metals enter the body in a variety of ways. They can come from silver amalgam fillings in the teeth (mercury), paint and other old structures (lead), conventionally-raised food, or water supplies (arsenic, manganese, lead). They can also come from a host of other environmental sources, including pesticides, herbicides, and other cleaning products. Many people have a history of working in industries that put them in contact with toxic components, such as printing, manufacturing, and certain fields involving arts and crafts. Frankly, it is hard to be alive at this point in history and not be exposed to heavy metals.

The longer I practice alternative therapies, the more aware I become of issues that prevent the body from healing. One of these is the issue we are discussing here: the presence of heavy metals in the body. When I evaluate patients, I am particularly interested in finding out if they have a history of working with or being exposed to heavy metals. I ask these types of questions: "Have you lived or worked on a farm that used sprays or pesticides? Have you worked in a factory where you were exposed to paint or other toxic fumes? Have you lived in smog or a polluted environment? For a time, I conducted a hair analysis to evaluate the presence of heavy metals in patients' bodies. However, my experience shows this test is not very accurate, so I no longer perform this test as a screen. Instead, I recommend and use the urine challenge test when measuring a patient's amount of heavy metals toxicity.

Urine Challenge Test

At our practice, one of the ways we recommend that all patients improve their health status is to be tested for the presence of heavy metals. Then, if we find they have a significant amount, we recommend they undergo chelation therapy. We recommend using a urine challenge test to evaluate the presence of heavy metals. This type of test is necessary for several reasons. Primarily, it is superior to other tests in determining your body's toxic load. If you had severe heavy metal poisoning—in fact, you could be on your deathbed—and had your blood tested for heavy metals, chances are the results would be normal. How can that be? Traditional blood tests are not accurate in these cases because heavy metals do not stay in your blood for long. Instead, they are absorbed into bones, fat tissues, and neurological tissues—especially the eyes. The key to measuring heavy metals is to force them into the blood and urine before taking the levels' measurement. The patient ingests a challenging agent that makes the metals stored in fat tissue and bone more soluble; then, this solution (the agent and the heavy metals it picks up) moves into the blood and urine.

This is how a urine challenge test works: A patient takes a chelating (removing) agent and then gives urine samples over a specific period of hours. The most commonly used chelating agents are EDTA and DMSA. A measured amount is given either orally or intravenously, depending on the patient's weight, age, and health, as well as on the heavy metal(s) being studied. Urine is then collected over six to twenty-four hours. The specimens are then sent to the laboratory for analysis and will provide a measurement of the amount of heavy metals. This analysis, therefore, gives a much better indication of a body's stored metals than a blood test does.

People who have significant toxic metal levels should seriously consider undergoing chelation therapy. Chelation therapy is the removal of heavy metals through urine and feces. Heavy metals are chelated from the tissues and into the waste stream. The technique introduces chelating agents, or chemical compounds that bind to metals and help remove them, to a patient's body. In the body, the chelating agent reacts with metal ions (such as lead, mercury, calcium, iron, and aluminum) and combines (that is, bonds) with the ions, forming a more chemically stable, non-soluble compound. Because the body cannot break down this non-soluble compound easily, it can be excreted (taking the metal along with it), through both the urinary and excretory systems.

Methods of Chelation

There are several chelation methods. First, chelation can be performed orally: patients ingest the chelating agents found in food or take it in pill form. Second, it can be performed through injecting the chelating agents intravenously. Third, chelation can also be performed topically— patients apply creams that contain chelating agents—or, fourth, it can even be done rectally. Chelation therapy is also used on individuals who have blocked blood vessels: chelation clears the vessels without using surgery, stents, or drugs. Further information on all four methods can be found later on in the chapter.

All forms of chelation, whether they are oral, topical, rectal, or intravenous, should be done under the supervision of a trained medical professional. This person can determine the amount of the chelating agent you need, the effectiveness of your treatment, and the necessary duration of treatment.

Foods as Oral Chelating Agents

The first step to preventing heavy metals accumulation—and, for some, the way to eliminate it—is through following a good diet. We have already discussed the importance of eating organic food that has not been exposed to toxic chemicals. However, there is another diet-related step you can take to improve your health. Many foods are good chelating agents for heavy metals. "Let your food be your medicine, and your medicine be your food," said Hippocrates. Deliberately including chelating foods in your diet is one way of making food into your medicine.

One of these potent medicinal foods is cilantro. Dr. David Williams published in the June 1998 issue of his newsletter, *Alternatives*, that cilantro can be used to detoxify the body and is the most interesting item to come down the pike, in this regard, in years. People have found cilantro can chelate heavy metals like mercury, aluminum, and lead from the body. In fact, some believe cilantro can cross the blood-brain barrier and actually remove heavy metals from the brain. Cilantro may be one of the most effective agents for this.

Cilantro, a member of the carrot family, is botanically known as *Coriandrum sativum*. The plant and leaves are called *cilantro*, while the seeds (used as a spice) are called *coriander*. The plant is often referred to as Mexican parsley or Chinese parsley. The leaves, which resemble those of flat-leaf parsley, are used for seasoning in Mexican and Asian dishes. Cilantro is sold fresh, in bunches, in most markets' produce sections. Avoid dried cilantro, which is pretty much worthless. Some people have a very strong aversion to the flavor and will object to even the smallest amount in a dish; even those who enjoy this herb agree that the flavor is definitely strong and pungent. However, even people with a very strong aversion to the cilantro flavor can overcome their dislike and still consume the plant. One way is to make pesto from the herb and use that pesto in pasta, bread, or egg dishes.

Dr. Yoshiaki Omura, Director of Medical Research at the Heart Disease Research Foundation, was conducting research on another topic and observed subjects had higher than normal levels of mercury in their urine after consuming Vietnamese soup, which had large amounts of cilantro in it. This was a good sign; higher mercury levels in urine mean mercury is being removed from the body. Dr. Omura followed up on this accidental finding and discovered that giving cilantro for several weeks to patients with mercury poisoning successfully eliminated this toxin from their bodies.

A large section of my family's garden is dedicated to cilantro, which we pick daily and add to soup, eggs, and salads. I am lucky in that my wife frequently makes us a delicious, authentic Vietnamese soup that contains a lot of cilantro. If you want to make this soup, I suggest trying my wife's recipe, which is listed below; you'll also find my "lazy man's" recipe. Other ways to enjoy cilantro are to put it in salads or, as I mentioned above, make a pesto. To make a pesto, use olive oil and either walnuts or Brazilian nuts; both these nuts are good sources of magnesium and zinc. Consider keeping a few pots of cilantro on your windowsill; that way, you will always have a fresh supply.

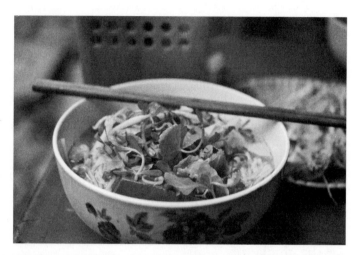

VIETNAMESE CHICKEN NOODLE SOUP

Broth:

   2 yellow **onions**, about 1 pound

   unpeeled 4-inch section fresh **ginger**

   1 organic free range **chicken** with skin on (around 4 lbs)

   4 set of **chicken bones** (carcasses)

   5 quarts **water**

   1½ tablespoons **salt**

   1 ounce of **rock sugar**

   2 tablespoons **coriander seeds**, *toasted in a dry skillet for about 1   minute until fragrant*

   1 stick of **cinnamon**

   1 large bunch of **cilantro**

Garnishes:

Cilantro, Bean sprouts, Thai basil, chiles, thinly sliced limes, cut into wedges

Make the pho broth:

1. Place the onions and ginger directly on the cooking grate of a medium-hot charcoal or gas grill or a gas stove with a medium flame, or on a medium-hot burner of an electric stove. Let the skin burn, using tongs to rotate onion and ginger occasionally and to grab and discard any flyaway onion skin.

2. Rinse the chicken and the chicken carcasses under cool water.

3. Remove and discard any loose pieces of fat from the chicken.

4. Put the chicken in the big pot filled with luke-warm water. Bring to a boil over high heat and then lower the heat to a gentle simmer. Use a ladle or large, shallow spoon to skim off any scum that rises to the top. Add the onions, ginger, salt, rock sugar, coriander seeds, cinnamon (put in a tea bag/tea ball), and cilantro and cook, uncovered, for 25 minutes, adjusting the heat if needed to maintain a gentle simmer.

At this point, the chicken is cooked; its flesh should feel firm yet still yield a bit to the touch. Use a pair of tongs to grab the chicken and transfer it to a large bowl. Flush the chicken with cold water and drain well, then it set aside for 15 to 20 minutes until it is cool enough to handle. Meanwhile, keep the broth at a steady simmer.

5. When chicken can be handled, use a knife to remove each breast half and the whole legs (thigh and drumstick). Don't cut these pieces further, or they'll lose their succulence. Set aside on a plate to cool completely, then cover with plastic wrap and refrigerate; bring to room temperature before assembling the bowls.

6. Put the carcasses in the pot and adjust the heat to simmer the broth gently for another 1½ hours. Avoid a hard boil, or the broth will turn cloudy.

7. Strain the broth through a fine-mesh sieve (or a coarse-mesh sieve lined with cheesecloth) positioned over a pot. Discard the solids. Use a ladle to skim as much fat from the top of the broth as you like. (To make this task easier, you can cool the broth, refrigerate overnight, lift off the solidified fat, and then reheat before continuing.) Taste and adjust the flavor with additional salt, and rock sugar. There should be about 4 quarts (16 cups) broth.

Assemble the pho bowls: If using dried noodles, cover them with hot tap water and let soak for 15 to 20 minutes, or until they are pliable and opaque. Drain in a colander. If using fresh rice noodles, untangle them, place in a colander, and rinse briefly under cold running water.

Cut the cooked chicken into slices about 1/4 inch thick, cutting the meat off the bone as necessary. If you don't want to eat the skin, discard it first. Set the chicken aside. Ready the yellow onion, scallions, cilantro, and pepper for adding to the bowls. Arrange the garnishes on a plate and put on the table.

For each bowl, place a portion of the noodles on a vertical-handle strainer (or mesh sieve) and dunk the noodles in the boiling water. As soon as they have collapsed and lost their stiffness (10 to 20 seconds), pull the strainer from the water, letting the water drain back into the pot. Empty the noodles into a bowl. If you like, once you have finished blanching the noodles, you can blanch the bean sprouts for 30 seconds. They should wilt slightly but retain some crunch. Drain and add to the garnishes.

Top each bowl of noodles with chicken, arranging the slices flat. Place a mound of cilantro in the center and then shower some scallion, yellow onion on top. Finish with a sprinkle of pepper and a teaspoon of fish sauce.

Raise the heat and bring the broth to a rolling boil. Do a final tasting and make any last-minute flavor adjustments. Ladle about 2 cups broth into each bowl, distributing the hot liquid evenly to warm all the ingredients. Serve immediately with the garnishes.

DR. KONDROT'S LAZY VIETNAMESE SOUP

Ingredients:

Organic **chicken broth**

Hand full of organic **cilantro**

Chopped organic **carrots**

Pinch of ground **chile pepper**

salt and **pepper** to taste

Preparation:

Heat all ingredients except cilantro

Add cilantro at the end and serve

Another food component that is good medicine is pectin. In her book *Prescription for Natural Healing*, Phyllis Balch reports that pectin helps diabetics, removes toxins and heavy metals, lowers cholesterol, and reduces the risk of gallstones. Pectin is in apples, bananas, citrus fruit rinds (lemons, oranges, and grapefruit), carrots, beets, cabbage, and okra. You can juice these foods, most likely getting some pectin in the pulp, and then you can add the pulp to muffins. Otherwise, there are several pectin supplements available.

Chlorella, which you can find in green algae, is also a mild chelator. Chlorella has a three-layered cell wall that contains cellulose microfibrils, which aid in heavy metal detoxification. You can obtain this all-important nutrient in supplements and in drinks from juice bars, or simply make a drink yourself by using chlorella powder, which is widely available.

Methionine is another naturally occurring chelating agent, one that supplies sulfur to the body. Methionine helps the body in heavy metal detoxification by increasing the production of cysteine and lecithin, which benefits the liver, and by protecting your kidneys. It is found in abundance in sesame seeds and other plant seeds.

In addition, fresh garlic is a good source of N-Acetyl-L-Cysteine (NAC), which increases the production of cysteine and glutathione, two powerful antioxidants that lessen the effects of heavy metals. If you find it hard to eat garlic, because of its pungent smell, you can take garlic supplements in capsule form.

Finally, milk thistle—a plant whose botanical name is silymarin—helps your liver detoxify. In the process, it also eliminates heavy metals. As a side benefit, milk thistle protects red blood cells' membranes.

Are you looking for help in incorporating all these agents into your diet? I met a wonderful organic chief, Sal Montezinos, in Naples, Florida, and the two of us are collaborating on a cookbook that will include recipes for curing eye disease. He has written an excellent raw organic cookbook, *Discovering Raw Alkaline Cuisine*, that can be downloaded from the internet at www.evolvewithflavor.com. This book is full of recipes created to help you on your journey to wellness and clear vision.

In the following passages, I describe the four major methods for chelating heavy metals from your body. Remember, however, that all these methods can also remove essential minerals. Because of this, it is important you take a good mineral supplement while undergoing chelation.

Oral Chelation

I used to think oral chelation (taking a chelating agent in capsule or pill form) had little value. Studies show that less than 10 percent of oral agents are absorbed into the body to help remove heavy metals. This is in comparison to a 100 percent absorption in intravenous therapy and 20 percent absorption via rectal administration. However, the oral agents are useful in preventative care; they will combine with the heavy metals found in most foods and prevent them from entering the body. Oral chelation is probably the best way to prevent additional toxins from entering the body. Anyone with a high toxic mineral load may need intravenous chelation instead. Remember the rain barrel analogy? When you have a disease, your rain barrel is filled with toxins. You need to do everything you can to prevent more toxins from entering your body.

There are many oral chelating agents on the market, but whichever you choose, you should chelate under a doctor's supervision. Be aware that all chelating agents will remove both toxic and essential minerals. Therefore, if you are taking oral agents, it is essential that you take supplemental minerals too. While one good thing is that the chelating agents have a much higher affinity (or attraction) to larger, more toxic minerals than to the smaller, essential minerals, *it is still important to monitor your minerals while undergoing chelation treatment.* This is one reason why I highly suggest people receiving chelation simultaneously receive the Myers' cocktail (a fortified intravenous vitamin mixture described in Chapter One). You can also consume Brazil nuts, which contain some of the highest amounts of zinc, selenium, and magnesium found in any food. Brazil nuts seem like a perfect snack for helping the body recover minerals during the chelation process.

Topical chelation

Amazingly, the application of a skin lotion can reverse years of changes in the eyes caused by heavy metal exposure! All aging changes in the body, wrinkled skin, hardening of the arteries, decrease in hearing, memory and vision are accelerated by toxins. A big contribution to our toxic exposure is heavy metals. In his *Second Opinion* newsletter (www.SecondOpinionNewsletter.com), Dr. Robert Rowen has recently reported on TD-DMPS, a skin lotion that is able to remove heavy metals from the body. Because your skin is rich in nerves, applying a lotion topically helps transport the DMPS (dimercapto-propane sulfonate) backward, first into the central nervous system and then into your brain and eyes.

Dr. Detrich Klinghard, a well-known alternative practitioner who treats autistic children poisoned by heavy metals, developed this treatment. To do so, he researched techniques of administering chelating agents without going the invasive, intravenous route. His method combines a chelating agent (DMPS) and glutathione: glutathione acts as a carrier, transporting the DMPS through the skin into the neurological tissues. This method eliminates intravenous treatment and there is some evidence that it is quite effective in the removal of heavy metals.

Thus, topical chelation is certainly a method to consider if you have difficulty with intravenous therapy or live a great distance from a chelation center.

Rectal Chelation

Rectal chelation is another option for the removal of heavy metals. Through this technique, about 20 percent of the chelation agent EDTA (ethylenediaminetetraacetic acid) is absorbed into the highly permeable rectal mucosa tissue. Rectal chelation can be a very effective option when intravenous therapy is not available or patients are looking for a more economical method of chelation delivery. One drawback, though, is that many patients develop loose stools using this method. In addition, just like oral or topical methods, patients employing this technique must also undertake a consistent replacement of essential minerals. In contrast, one advantage of intravenous chelation is that most chelating doctors end such a treatment with a mineral boost that helps patients keep a healthy level of minerals.

Intravenous Chelation

Intravenous (IV) chelation is superior to oral, topical, and rectal chelation in its effectiveness. When you undertake IV chelation, 100 percent of the chelating agent will enter your body, supplying you with the maximum dose and targeting the heavy metals that are locked into your bones, fat, and neurological tissues. I also recommend IV chelation since it must be done under medical supervision: the doctor overseeing the therapy will ensure that the proper amount of chelating agent is administered and that trace minerals are replaced regularly. This will greatly lessen the chance of patients developing mineral deficiencies. You can find a chelation practitioner through the American College for the Advancement of Medicine (www.acam.org). This organization of MDs and other professionals is committed to the use of chelation therapy. One of its members can assist you with proper testing and treatment.

So, fill up on the good stuff, clean out the bad stuff, and get ready to add even more tools to your vision-healing toolbox.

CHAPTER TWO NOTES

Websites
Compare and purchase water filters:
www.purewaterproducts.com

How to compost:
www.compostinstructions.com

Pure salt:
www.himalasalt.com

Cilantro as a Mercury Chelator:
Significant mercury deposits in internal organs following the removal of dental amalgam, and development of pre-cancer on the gingiva and the sides of the tongue and their represented organs as a result of inadvertent exposure to strong curing light (used to solidify synthetic dental filling material) and effective treatment: a clinical case report, along with organ representation areas for each tooth.

Omura, Y., Shimotsuura, Y., Fukuoka, A., Fukuoka, H., and T. Nomoto. *Acupuncture and Electrotherapeutics Research* 21, no. 2 (Apr. - Jun. 1996): 133-60.

CHAPTER 3

Relaxation

Assuming that you do all of the things I have recommended up to this point to achieve better health—change your diet, keep yourself hydrated, and maintain adequate mineral intake—a critical part of the puzzle is still missing. If this puzzle piece is not addressed, it really does not matter how vigilant you are with your diet and hydration; you are not going to regain your health completely. This next piece, or step, is balancing your autonomic nervous system. The autonomic nervous system has two parts: the sympathetic and the parasympathetic. It is essential that these two systems are in balance to achieve health.

The sympathetic nervous system is what produces the "fight or flight" response in people. For example, when a grizzly bear chases you in the woods and you are running for your life, certain physiological changes take place in your body. Your pupils dilate and your heart races. Your body does not digest food, nor does it heal; instead, it uses all its energy and resources to survive. In a sympathetic state, all your body's physiological healing processes stop.

Unfortunately, most of us live in a state of constant sympathetic nervous system arousal. There are many ways we can become stressed and thereby awaken our sympathetic nervous system. Sources of stress can be emotional, physical, or mental. For example, suppose your doctor tells you that you have macular degeneration, you are going to go blind, and nothing can be done. This diagnosis and prognosis would stress you greatly—just at a time when you need all your healing resources fully available.

Sometimes stress factors are less personal. For example, suppose you turn on the television and listen to the news. That will usually be enough to put you in a sympathetic state. When you are in this state, even little things irritate you; if somebody cuts you off in traffic or the alarm clock goes off, you jump. This response is physiological. Unless you practice relaxation techniques, you have no control over the way your body responds. Most of us have been in the sympathetic state for so long that our sympathetic nervous systems are burned out and we have nothing left but real fatigue. This sets the stage for the development of chronic diseases.

Our goal is to have our body in a parasympapthetic state. This is a state of relaxation. Our heart rate and breathing slow down. Our blood pressure is lowered and digestion improves. Most importantly the natural healing abilities of the body can take place while we are in a parasympathetic state.

WE ALL HAVE A PERSONAL GRIZZLY BEAR

Let's get back to that grizzly bear. Some time ago, when I was in Montana, I was giving a talk about relaxation and balancing the autonomic nervous system in Montana. I had everyone's attention when I started to talk about grizzly bears and the fight or flight response to stress. The reason everyone was so interested in my remark is because there are a many grizzly bears in Montana. Every store sells pepper spray, which is reported to be the best way to stop a charging grizzly bear. It is supposed to be even more effective than a high-powered rifle. You can shoot a grizzly bear several times and he will keep charging, but one shot of pepper spray to the bear's face and he will turn around. No Montanan will leave home without a can of pepper spray. That's what the experts say, at least. However, an editorial in a local Montana newspaper recently challenged the pepper spray defense. The article's author says you have to be a real fool to believe that one shot of pepper spray will truly stop a thousand-pound, charging grizzly bear; the only way pepper spray will help is if you use it to spray yourself in your face. You will be in so much pain you will be happy the grizzly bear ends your life! The author also jokes that the only other option, if you've got pepper spray, is to spray your companion; when he becomes disabled by the spray, *run*, and let the grizzly bear attack him.

Seriously, though, we need good ways to get rid of these "grizzly bears" that represent our fears and put us into sympathetic states.

BALANCING TECHNIQUES FOR THE NERVOUS SYSTEM

There are many ways to balance your autonomic nervous system. The method does not have to be complicated, but it does need to be consistent. There are two components to finding balance; the first is to learn what we call the "relaxation response." This allows you to relax or remain relaxed even when something stressful enters your world. This relaxation is achieved by a daily practice of meditation, relaxation, prayer, and/or exercise. The second component is to learn how to relax the sympathetic nervous system quickly when it is aroused.

Use Light to Balance

One of my favorite ways to balance the autonomic nervous system is through the powerful and rapid method of light therapy. We have already talked about the sympathetic and the parasympathetic parts of the autonomic nervous system. In light therapy, the sympathetic nervous system is represented by red energy and the parasympathetic by blue. We all know that it can be very relaxing to walk outside and gaze up at the blue sky on a nice, clear, sunny day. Looking at the color blue in the sky relaxes your autonomic nervous system. Similarly, looking at blue water when you're at the beach or on a boat seems to be very relaxing. The reason looking at blue seems this way is that this form of color therapy very quickly balances the autonomic nervous system.

To give you an idea of how quickly you can balance your autonomic nervous system, I'd like to share a personal experience with you. I first found out about light therapy when I was giving a lecture in Santa Fe, New Mexico. I had just arrived; I was jet-lagged and I had some anxiety about my presentation. Some of the people at the conference were conducting autonomic nervous system evaluations by measuring their subjects' peripheral vision fields. If your peripheral vision is restricted, that means your sympathetic nervous system is aroused. This arousal restricts your visual field because, when you are running and the grizzly bear is chasing you (for example), you need tunnel vision to stay focused on your escape. A restricted visual field means you are feeling fear. In this case, my fear was not because of any grizzly bear but was because of my performance anxiety. During the test my colleagues gave me, they also found my eye movements were kind of jumpy; a couple of other parameters were off, too.

My associates provided me with ten minutes of light therapy. This means that for ten minutes, I just looked at a certain spectrum of light. Then my colleagues measured the same areas—my visual field and the jumpy quality of eye movements—again. Everything had improved dramatically. That experience convinced me that light therapy works very quickly.

Blood Exposed to Light

Dr. Tina Karu, a Russian investigator, is known for her work in dynamic light therapy. Her research includes a procedure in which she takes blood out of a patient's body and passes it through a glass tube. While the blood is passing through the tube, she exposes it to different light spectrums. After this, she re-injects the blood into the patient. Then, she measures physiological changes in the body, such as blood pressure and heart rate, as well as neuroendocrine, hypothalamus gland, and pituitary gland functions. It was determined that all values improved with light therapy. Light therapy is not only very effective; it is also free and natural. To take advantage of it, just go outside.

Many of us are already responsive to light's impact. We demonstrate this when we choose to wear certain colors. Often, we dress in specific colors because we are attempting to balance our autonomic nervous system. Wearing red is not bad. Some people are nutritionally depleted and their autonomic system is burned out; they actually need red energy to inject some life into themselves.

Breath

Another way to help balance the autonomic nervous system is through practicing slow, deep breathing. Whenever you are upset and anxious, take a deep breath.

Breath is one part of the autonomic nervous system people can control. We cannot tell our heart rate to slow down or convince our blood pressure to drop to 120 over 80, but we can control our breathing. Breathing is actually the link between the sympathetic and the parasympathetic nervous systems. When breathing is going on unconsciously, it is part of the parasympathetic system; when we focus on it, or bring it under conscious control, then it becomes part of the sympathetic system.

In addition to breath, positive affirmation, prayer, and relaxation practices can all help our autonomic nervous system. I am convinced that when people who are anxious and focused on their diseases come into my office, they really need to begin to control the sympathetic nervous system as part of their healing process. They can change their diet, they can drink plenty of water, and they can take zinc, but if they don't shift that autonomic nervous system and make it less stressed, they are not going to see real improvement in their health. Most of the time, the most important step you can take for your healing is to balance your autonomic nervous system.

One New Mexican patient attended my three-day program for vision healing and had an admirable change in his attitude as a result. He had spent several years in a very negative environment, being tested and treated by an eye doctor who repeatedly said that nothing could be done to improve this patient's vision. However, the patient persevered, and, after the program he had an improvement in both his vision and his attitude. "Dr. Kondrot," he told me, "I no longer have macular *degeneration*. I have macular *regeneration*."

Music to Relax

Another way to relax and help balance the autonomic nervous system is by listening to music. Artists have recorded many excellent CDs of music for relaxation. One of my favorites is the series of relaxation music by Australian artist Tony O'Connor. His instrumental music is amazing in its ability to quiet the mind and relax the body.

Coincidentally, another musician named O'Connor has influenced me and, to this day, still helps me to relax. He's Mark O'Connor, a famous American fiddle player. I enjoy playing the fiddle to relax, and every year I attend Mark's fiddle camp in Eastern Tennessee. Even if you are not musically gifted, learning to play an instrument can help you to relax. I also believe that when you play your own instrument, you will be attracted to melodies and tunes that are particularly healing for you.

While we may have experienced music's power to help us relax or to invigorate us, there is not much hard evidence about how it works. The good news about this is that we don't need to know how music's relaxation capabilities work in order to apply music therapy to our lives. We do know a few things about music and relaxation for sure, however. One is that we listen to and make music by using the right side of our brain. This is the area of the brain we know is more intuitive, creative, and holistic; it does not separate things into components. So, when we listen to music, we can just get swept away by the effect of all the instruments (including voices) blending together. Rarely do we try to pick out individual instruments and notes; when we do that, we are probably "listening with the left side" of our brains. Music has the power to distract us from unpleasant or worrisome thoughts; it can shift our sympathetic state to a parasympathetic one. Once we have shifted our state, we can access many more internal resources. We can solve problems and begin to heal. In this more receptive state, you will draw even more information and resources to yourself, so you will have a lot more to work with in the healing process.

The second way music helps us is that it shifts us from a mental state to a more emotional state. Such a state may seem sort of "empty" or floating, which is in direct contrast to the fuller state of anxiety, contributed to by a profusion of thoughts. Finally, listening to music may transport us to other times and places. An aria might remind us of a time in Italy when we went to the opera, while a lullaby might recall our own childhood or our children's childhoods. As long as these memories we recall are pleasant, we are still doing ourselves a lot of good with music.

Everyone has preferences regarding the type or types of music they enjoy. (Did you ever take an automobile trip with a teenager before iPods were invented?) We probably like different types of music at different times in our lives, at different times of the day, and even on different days of the week. For relaxation purposes, however, studies show that certain types of music excel. These types include music with a tempo of sixty beats per minute (like a heartbeat), music with low tones, and musical compositions rendered by stringed instruments, rather than brass or percussion. If you ever have the chance to listen to Samuel Barber's *Adagio for Strings*, you can hear some lovely music that has all these characteristics.

I have selected one of my favorite opera arias, "Nessun Dorma," to introduce my talk radio show, *Healthy Vision*. This aria is about overcoming extreme obstacles to achieve a successful outcome. Some of the words in the aria are "*Vincerò, vincerò,*" which translate to "I will conquer, I will conquer!" In turn, it is my goal to help you conquer your vision loss! Each time I hear this aria, I become inspired all over again. It always elevates me to a higher level of enthusiasm.

Relaxation: The Ultimate Empowerment

Whether you decide to relax by using music, meditation, yoga, or another method, there is one important thing to remember. The more often and the more quickly you can reach a relaxed state, the easier you will find it to relax when you are confronted by upsetting thoughts or situations. The idea is to build up neural pathways that prompt you to relax regardless of what is going on. We all have our personal "grizzlies" and stress triggers, but few of them are really going to attack or kill us. It's more likely that we are attacking and killing ourselves because we stay in hyper-aroused states when there is no real threat.

Think back to the last time you were traveling and your flight was delayed. Travelers respond to these types of delays in several predictable ways. A few people will always engage airline personnel in an argument or express their feelings vocally. Many people "check out," slumping in their seats and internalizing their frustration. Quite a few grab their cell phones and express their frustration to their loved ones or colleagues. After all, they are going to be late. How awful is that? Finally, some people pick up a book or begin listening to relaxing music while they wait the delay out. They may even have some soothing self-talk about how all things happen for the best; maybe they will avoid an accident or meet an interesting person due to this delay. The important thing to note here is that everyone will eventually get on the plane at the same time, but during the waiting period some will have done some real damage to their health, while others will have practiced relaxation.

The lesson in the above example is that while you cannot always control what happens to you, you can always determine your attitude or response. This knowledge is actually very empowering, since many people find feeling helpless (for example, thinking, "The plane is delayed, and there is nothing I can do about it.") is a huge contributor to stress. But, you see, you are never helpless; you always have the power to choose your response to any challenge presented by life.

Some of you reading this book may feel discouraged when you realize that you have been eating junk, you have not drinking the proper amount or the best type of water, or maybe you have even given in to hopelessness because of a diagnosis you have received. Well, turn those thoughts around. Be grateful that today you can start making changes that will benefit you for the rest of your life. Wherever you are is the right place to begin. Just be sure you do begin!

CHAPTER THREE NOTES

Gottlieb, Raymond L., and Larry B. Wallace. "Syntonic Phototherapy." *Photomedicine and Laser Surgery* 28, no. 4 (2010): 449–452.

Karu, Tina. "The Science of Low Power Laser Therapy." *Informa Healthcare*, 1998. London.

Puccini, Giacomo. *Turandot.* Perf. Luciano Pavarotti and Joan Sutherland. London Philharmonic Orchestra, 1990, compact disc. Label: Decca, ASIN: B0000041Q3

Rowen, Robert Jay. "Ultraviolet Blood Irradiation Therapy (Photo-Oxidation)." *International Journal of Biosocial and Medical Research* 14, no. 2 (1996): 115-32.

Move More, See Better

Everyone knows that exercise is important to good health. However, exercising becomes even more important for people as they age; it is also important for anyone with a chronic or serious eye condition. Exercise's benefits can be compared to good nutrition's; while exercising will be good for your overall health, it will also directly affect and improve your ability to see.

You may be wondering how that can happen. We have two types of vision: visual acuity and functional vision. Basically, visual acuity is a measurement that shows how well you can see when you are focused on an eye chart, a light, or some other target. Functional vision may be quite different from acuity; it is the indicator of how well we see when we are using our eyes as they were intended to be used normally. In other words, "functional vision" means what you're doing when your eyes are simply responding to your environment, not seeking out specific targets to look at.

Functional vision relies a lot on three functions: peripheral vision, scanning ability, and, believe it or not, balance and posture. Therefore, exercises that improve these functions will improve your functional vision, thereby improving your ability to see—regardless of your eyeglasses prescription. We will discuss the difference between visual acuity and function in more detail in Chapter 5, when we talk about vision therapy. My goal in this chapter, especially if you are a person who does not exercise regularly, is to introduce you to some forms of exercise that you may not have considered before. Many wonderful workouts can be fun, worked into your regular schedule, and done from home.

THE TRAMPOLINE

Remember when you were a kid and jumped up and down, and up and down, on a trampoline? You thought it was just fun, and it was. Yet this fun form of movement also has tremendous benefits for both the immune system and vision. It also has a new name; we call what happens when adults jump on trampolines "rebounding." Using a rebounder (a small trampoline) is a wonderful option for everyone, especially seniors or folks recuperating from accidents or injuries. It's also excellent exercise for those who have been sedentary and are just starting an exercise program.

Using a trampoline or rebounding is an easy and fun way to obtain many health benefits right in your own home or backyard. You can choose between family-sized trampolines and personally-sized rebounders. Smaller trampolines are safer than the larger ones (which measure eight to fourteen feet), due to the former's close proximity to the ground.

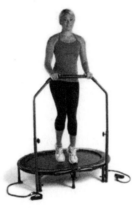

If you have balance issues, you can buy a rebounder with rails to hold onto until you get your "flying legs." These items are quite reasonably priced, ranging from $99 to $500. The main rebounder variable seems to be durability. The cheaper ones wear out or tear more quickly. If price matters to you, I suggest you buy a cheaper one and see whether you will actually use it or not. Trade up to a more expensive one when you decide to work rebounding into your life on a regular basis.

A few of rebounding's benefits include gaining a better sense of balance, achieving an enhanced sense of rhythm, and finding the ability to experience both sides of the body, or achieving bilateral awareness. These benefits are invaluable in helping to coordinate eye movements or to overcome the tendency to use your dominant eye (or side of the body). When you are on the trampoline, your left side and right side must bounce in unison, and you must maintain a steady rhythm throughout the body. Few other activities demand such a rhythm. Using a trampoline forces the brain to function bilaterally, which results in improved bilateral motor skill development and improved vision.

Rebounding is good for anyone who is reluctant to begin physical activities. Because it seems like play, even those of us who fear the gym or are averse to workouts may find ourselves taking little breaks throughout the day to jump. No special clothes or equipment are needed, either. Jumping on a trampoline is easy; it offers immediate success and a sense of accomplishment. It promotes many other health benefits, including a feeling of exhilaration, as described in the next section.

Increases Lymphatic Circulation

The body's lymphatic system is a network of vessels. The vessels transport nutrients and drain toxic products from tissues. The network does not contain its own pumping mechanism. Instead, it relies on external pressure, including breathing and muscular contractions, to propel its contents through a system of one-way lymphatic valves. Using a trampoline helps the lymphatic system eliminate toxins because you increase the gravitational pull on your body as you bounce.

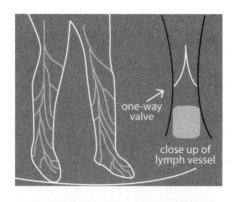

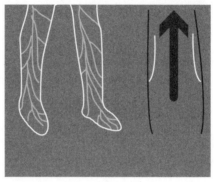

Benefits for Glaucoma Patients

I also like to recommend rebounding as an exercise method for patients with glaucoma. In addition to providing exercise-related benefits, stimulating the lymphatic system has a pressure-lowering effect on the eye.

Increased Bone Density

You can strengthen your bones, just as you can strengthen your muscles, through moderate physical activity. Studies show that people who exercise at least three times a week have a higher mineral content in their bones, which correlates to much stronger bones. Improving bone density also reduces the chance of debilitating fractures and deformities associated with osteoporosis.

Low Impact Exercise is Easy on the Joints

The main disadvantage of another form of exercise, jogging, is the physical stress it places on the lower limbs and feet. In contrast, using the trampoline takes off up to 80 percent of the stress on your weight-bearing joints. Spending ten to twenty minutes using the trampoline is equal to spending about thirty minutes jogging. Because the trampoline mat absorbs some of the impact's shock on each jump, there is no strain on the joints. When repeated, this low-impact exercise builds and strengthens the bones and muscles, resulting in increased toning, better balance, improved coordination, and stronger posture.

Heart and Circulation

The action of bouncing up and down against the pull of gravity strengthens all the body's system. Jumping on a trampoline is considered to be one of the most beneficial aerobic exercises ever developed. The heart itself is strengthened, due to the increase in heart rate caused by jumping. Jumping also increases circulation by releasing energy and pumping oxygen into the brain. (Later on, in Chapter 9, we will discuss the importance of sufficient oxygenation to good vision.)

Better Mood

Jumping on a trampoline is exercise in disguise. It uses almost every muscle, specifically those in the stomach, arms, and legs. Muscles are toned, fat is burned, and metabolism is increased. All this makes a trampoline a successful tool for weight loss. Working out on a trampoline rejuvenates both the body and the mind. It increases endorphins, producing positive, mood-enhancing natural chemicals. This helps overcome negativity and depression, and helps people become happier, more positive individuals.

Weight Loss

Finally, a study conducted by researchers at the University of California, San Diego, found that using a trampoline can contribute to weight loss. "Exercise on a miniature trampoline is not significantly different from treadmill running or stationary bicycling in increasing fitness and decreasing body fat in overweight women."

Improve all your systems, your vision, your balance, and coordination, and improve your overall health, with a tool that costs under $100? It almost seems to good to be true. I suggest you give it a try.

DANCING

Since we have been discussing rhythm, we need to talk about dancing. Dancing is another way to improve coordination, balance, peripheral vision, and eye-to-foot coordination. It also can improve social skills. Ballroom dancing is a great method. So are the many new forms of rhythmic movement, such as Zumba, a fitness program in which groups move to quick and upbeat Latin tunes. The program's official slogan is "Ditch the workout, and join the party." Zumba is definitely high energy and upbeat. YouTube.com has several videos that provide an orientation to this activity. A quick Internet search will lead you to many DVDs you can purchase, so you can get started with Zumba in your own home. Alternatively, you join a class; they are popping up everywhere. If having the right attire and shoes is important to you, you can find many shopping resources online. Again, the most important thing to do is to get started. Dance with a partner, alone, or in a class. Whatever keeps you motivated and moving is the right method for you.

Can Dance Lower Your Eye Pressure?

Peter Abilogu, an African Dance professor, recently completed our three-day *Restore Your Vision* program. He entered the program with a twenty-year history of *glaucoma*. Over the last couple of years, he has lost a great deal of vision. He has a keen interest in alternative treatments, particularly dance. Some Africans believe that when people dance in bare feet, they become connected to the earth's healing energy. The dance movements, along with the music, produce vibrations that help heal the body.

During the program, Peter underwent our standard treatments of microcurrent therapy, syntonic light therapy, and homeopathy. After two days of treatment, his eye pressures were reduced from twenty-three to seventeen. (Normal pressure is under twenty.) Because of the extensive damage to his optic nerve (He could only see the big E with his right eye and could barely see light with his left eye.) I believed his pressure needed to be even lower than seventeen. Peter and I decided to do an experiment to see if African dance could lower the pressure. This is where the fun began!

After dancing for one hour, his pressures were reduced to thirteen in both eyes. Peter told me his pressures had never been that low. We checked his vision and realized he was seeing five lines better on the eye chart. In addition, his visual field had expanded!

Scholars have published several articles on the pressure-lowering effects of exercise. I believe that dance, especially types of dance in which the dancer is grounded on the earth, might have an even greater affect on lowering pressure. Dr. Steven Sinatra, an integrative cardiologist, believes that "earthing" (or "grounding") may be the most important health recommendation he's given in his last thirty years of practice. Simply put, earthing reconnects the human body with the energy that's naturally present in the ground we all walk on.

The practice of using the earth's energy involves grounding a person to the earth, much like grounding an electrical current. When grounding occurs, electrons flow freely back and forth between the earth and the human body. This helps detoxify the harmful electromagnetic energy that accumulates in the body. Lastly, grounding helps balance the autonomic nervous system. So, how do you begin grounding? Walk barefoot on the earth. Take your shoes off at home and let your feet touch the concrete floor. If you can't go barefoot, eliminate rubber-soled shoes and wear leather. Rubber is an insulator; in contrast, leather conducts the earth's current.

Grounding might also help improve the affects of microcurrent therapy in eye disease treatment. We are asking patients to begin to test this by alternating microcurrent treatments between non-grounded and grounded states. How can you change states during your microcurrent treatment? Go outside. Simply take off your shoes and place your bare feet either on concrete or on the ground, and give yourself your treatment. In the next section, you'll learn about types of movements to help vision that are traditionally done outside.

TAI CHI AND QI GONG

Perhaps something a bit slower than rebounding or dancing, and something more meditative, would best suit your ability and temperament. Although Tai Chi started out as a martial art, most of today's practitioners teach it because of its health benefits. Tai Chi's set of exercises is part of the 4,000-year-old system of traditional medicine practiced in China. When it is practiced alongside the complementary Qi Gong (pronounced "chee gong"), the two form a synergistic relationship, which results in an incredibly effective health maintenance system.

While Qi Gong is sometimes called the new yoga, the practice dates back thousands of years to ancient China. The word "qi" (or "chi") means "life force" or "vital energy of the body," while "gong" means "a skill that is cultivated through steady practice." Qi Gong is specifically designed to cultivate the body's vital energy, using that energy to heal and strengthen every system throughout the body. In other words, Qi Gong involves working with energy to strengthen and cleanse the body.

If you cannot find a Tai Chi or Qi Gong class at your local senior center or community center, you can learn these techniques at home. Many DVDs are available online and instructional programs can be found everywhere. I particularly liked the online program at taichiforseniorsvideo.com because it is geared to beginners of any age, not just to seniors, and because it combines Tai Chi and Qi Gong. Here is some descriptive information from that website:

> *Most forms of exercise dissipate your energy and make you tired and hyper at the same time! Our form of Chi Kung [Qi Gong]/Tai Chi accumulates energy and leaves you refreshed and relaxed when you finish. The graceful, slow speed of our styles, coupled with an emphasis on deep breathing and mental focus, creates balance, flexibility, and calmness, which relieves stress and allows for the integration of your mind and body.*

For Qi Gong fans, Lee Holden's beginner program strengthens the entire body by encouraging it to follow its natural energy flow (www.exercisetoheal.com). Here is what Lee says about his work:

You'll learn the five "postures of power," and enjoy a series of standing meditations that will restore your internal balance. Filmed on the banks of a beautiful canyon stream, this is a delightful way to restore harmony to your body, mind, and spirit. Qi Gong mirrors the movements of nature, especially the fluidity of water. Qi Gong Flow for Beginners trains the body to be more relaxed, creating a sense of effortless ease. You'll find yourself slipping into the moment as the body circulates newfound internal energy. Although the body is moving, the mind remains centered, creating a dynamic balance between tranquility and internal strength.

WHOLE-BODY VIBRATIONAL TRAINING

Does exercising make you think of hours in the gym, watching boring news programs, or of being wired to the music in your headphones as you cycle, walk on a treadmill, or do other time-consuming and repetitive motions? Well, things have changed. In an effort to make exercise more appealing and efficient, people have created a new exercise concept called vibrational training. Vibrational training combines voluntary movement with electrical vibration.

The result is that the body moves in three dimensions and each muscle group is worked rapidly and effectively.

The class of equipment called vibrational trainers includes a variety of products. Vibration trainers transmit waves of energy throughout the body, activating muscle contractions between twenty-five and fifty times per second. This enhances overall performance in sessions as short as fifteen minutes a day, three times a week. In addition to the increased contraction speed, the vibration's influence ensures that more muscle fibers are activated than in normal, conscious muscle contractions. Doing this type of exercise uses muscles more efficiently, thus increasing bone density, balance, and muscle power. Compared with traditional training methods, vibrational training equipment helps people achieve greater results and increase hormonal production in much less time.

While there are many brands of vibrational trainers to choose from, I prefer the Power Plate® brand because it is widely used by many alternative doctors and because it is of extremely high quality. The Power Plate® comes in several sizes and speeds and is a bit of an investment; be prepared to spend upwards of $2,000 on one. You may be able to find a gym or spa near you where you can use the equipment as part of your membership. This could be a good permanent solution, or a way to experience the machine and decide whether it might be a good investment.

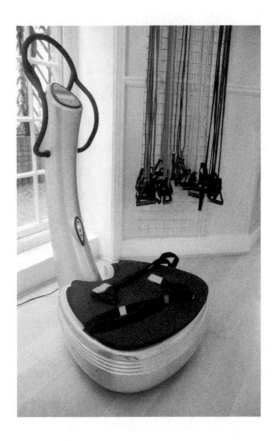

Here is some more detailed information about the Power Plate® from the manufacturer (www.powerplate. com/us/products):

Acceleration Training with Power Plate® machines creates instability in the human body, as with each vibration the body is forced to perform reflexive muscle actions multiple times per second. Furthermore, these contractions must work in multiple dimensions as the Power Plate® machines actually oscillate in all three planes, exactly as the human body is designed to do. The net result is an incredible improvement in strength and power. Training on Power

Plate® equipment offers a host of benefits, ranging from an immediate improvement in blood circulation to a variety of other measurable outcomes. [These include] increased muscle strength and flexibility, improved range of motion, decreased cellulite, increased bone mineral density, reduced pain and soreness, and faster recovery. Power Plate® is the ultimate wellness solution for all ages, lifestyles, and physical abilities.

One of the most important features of this type of workout is its efficiency. A whole host of benefits can be yours after investing just a minimum amount of time. This combination makes such exercise valuable. Statistics show that most in-home workout equipment just gathers dust in garages, while many people who become gym members fail to attend sessions after the first few months. Exercising fifteen minutes a day, three times per week is something most of us can commit to doing. Who knows? You might even be able to do more.

SUMMARY

We have reviewed several ways to get your body moving: from fast to slow, from stationary to bouncing, from using internal to external rhythm, and from expensive to almost free. I hope you have found a way that suits you and that you will begin to add one or more of these approaches to your plan to regain or retain your health.

CHAPTER FOUR NOTES

Marcus, Daniel. "The Effect of Exercise on Intraocular Pressure." *Investigative Ophthalmology and Visual Science* 9, no.10 (October 1970): 753-757.

Conclusion: The study found a statistically significant decrease in pressure during jogging and measured that decrease as a two- to five-point drop in pressure thirty minutes after exercise.

Natis, Konstantinos, et al. "Aerobic Exercise and Intraocular Pressure in Normotensive and Glaucoma Patients." *BMC Ophthalmology* 9, no. 6 (13 Aug. 2009).

Conclusion: In normal eyes of sedentary subjects who engage in moderate to heavy exercise for three months, a consistent decrease in pressure occurs (on the order of twelve points). As for glaucoma patients, regardless of the anti-glaucoma medication instilled, they still benefited from the aerobic exercise since they all had a post-exercise reduction of pressure. Short-term studies show it may improve blood flow to the retina and optic nerve as well.

Vision Therapy

Vision therapy, a type of physical therapy for the eyes and brain, is a highly effective, non-surgical treatment for many common visual problems, such as lazy eyes, crossed eyes, double vision, and convergence insufficiency. Vision therapy can also help with some reading and learning disabilities. Many patients who have been told, "It's too late" or "You'll have to learn to live with it" have benefited from vision therapy for their eye conditions.

In this book, we are going to talk about a different aspect of vision. Most people are familiar with the aspect called "visual acuity," which is the ability to see letters on an eye chart. We need to take that acuity and turn it into "functioning vision." In other words, this means taking the visual acuity you have and using it in your environment for daily activities (such as reading, watching television, doing crossword puzzles, and so forth) with improved functional capacity.

Even if you have good visual acuity (meaning you can see the letters on an eye chart during an eye exam), you might not have good visual function. There are three basic visual skills we can evaluate. The first one is called *pursuit*. It is the ability to follow an object in space with the eyes; you follow a car, a bird, or some other object that is creating some type of movement. The second skill is called *saccadic movement*; it is the ability to change visual fixation. If I am looking at something on one side, and I hear a noise on the other side, I will quickly change my focal point and look toward the noise. Poor saccadic ability can be observed when you overshoot; you look too far to one side and then you bounce back to the target. You lose that ability to fixate precisely on the spot where you want to look. Finally, the third visual skill is to be able to *fixate in space*, or to be able to hold your attention on an object that is remaining still.

We have many, many sophisticated vision therapy exercises and task evaluations. Typically, what we do in vision therapy is much like what a doctor does during any medical evaluation: first, we try to determine what the symptoms are; second, we try to determine which goals are realistic for a given situation. For example, if a patient has macular degeneration and vision problems, he might have problems backing that big RV he owns up or out of his driveway. When he backs it out, he might hit a pole and cause his vehicle some damage. So, because of macular degeneration, he would have a visual problem that would result in him hitting a pole with his RV. Because this patient knows it is unlikely he will regain perfect vision, he needs a solution that will allow him to maneuver his RV safely.

Our eyesight is more than just visual acuity. It is a function of the brain and something that we all have the ability to do. Recovering this ability is a matter of training your brain to see what's in front of you instead of seeing distortions. However, this is a complex issue; if your body's autonomic nervous system is out of balance, correcting it will involve re-balancing many systems, organs, and processes.

The therapy we offer, called *vision therapy* or *vision training*, involves using certain exercises and techniques that can dramatically improve your visual functions. Remember, our main goal for anybody who has an eye problem is twofold: first, we want to improve acuity, which measures what the person can see on the eye chart; second, we want to improve function. After working with some of these techniques, many patients can see two or three lines better on the eye chart. However, sometimes they come back and tell us, "I am reading better, but I still have trouble functioning in daily life." The goal at our practice goal is to have both acuity and function working as well as possible.

Personally, I think it is more important to have good function than acuity. I can tell stories about patients who have 20/20 vision but can't function. They have headaches, have trouble seeing signs, or cannot retain information after reading. In contrast, sometimes we see patients who have trouble seeing the big "E" on the eye chart but have no limitation in function. They are functioning fine, doing all of the daily activities that they enjoy. Which is a better state to be in? Personally, I would rather have poor acuity and better function. Functionality does not have to be linked with acuity. So, one of our goals in vision training is to introduce therapies and exercises that improve function.

THE BATES METHOD FOR SELF-TRAINING TO IMPROVE VISION

In the following passages, I describe some of the easiest and most effective techniques anywhere in this book—and they can be done at home, without any special equipment or any fees. You will find it really easy to build these eye routines into many other parts of your day. You can practice them when driving or riding in a car, waiting in any type of experience, or sitting in almost any room of your home at any time in the day. It's that easy! The important thing is to make a commitment to these techniques and practice them. I know you will want to do so after reading the rest of this chapter.

Eye Doctors Can Harm You

No doubt you are familiar with the process of having your eyesight tested. You sit in a darkened room. The examiner uses a very large piece of equipment to gaze at the inner parts of your eye, looking through the pupil (the black part in the center of the eye). To make the examination go more smoothly, the doctor puts drops in your eyes to make both pupils expand, or dilate. This usually makes it very difficult for you to focus on anything with clarity. Prior to putting the drops in your eyes, the examiner will ask you to read an eye chart. The chart has several lines of letters. As you move from top to bottom, each line gets smaller. Depending on how many lines you can read, the doctor can determine how to express the accuracy of your vision. This expression is done in terms of a fraction, with 20 as the denominator. If your vision is 20/20, it is considered perfect. What 20/20 actually means is that at a distance of 20 feet, you can see what test subjects could see at 20 feet. If your vision is 20/40, this means that at a distance of 20 feet, you can see what these people saw at 40 feet. If your vision is 20/100, this means the test subjects could see at 100 feet what you can see at 20 feet. A score of 20/200 or greater means you are legally blind. After the examiner takes your measurement, he or she will give you a prescription for "corrective" lenses—either glasses or contact lenses—to wear. This is in order to bring your vision as close as possible to 20/20.

William Bates

Perhaps the idea that people can reverse vision problems is new to you. It is not, however, a new idea in history. Important contributions to the topic came from William Bates, who was born in Newark, New Jersey, in 1860. He was a well-trained ophthalmologist who, in addition to his practice, lectured and wrote articles. In his book, *Perfect Sight Without Glasses*, Bates explains his simple but revolutionary theory about vision. The foundation of his theory revolves around four statements, as summarized by Peter Mansfield in his excellent book, *The Bates Method*, and reprinted here:

- Normal sight is inherently variable.
- Defective sight can get better as well as worse.
- Poor sight and eye disease are intimately related.
- Eyesight is an important indicator of mental, emotional, and physical health.

I'd like to discuss Bates' tenets one at a time. The first—the idea that "normal sight is inherently variable"— points to one of the greatest flaws in our traditional testing protocol. When we perform eye exams, we eye doctors figuratively "freeze" people in time and space, taking measurements of something that, by its nature, is fluid and constantly changing. Using an earlier version of the very same ophthalmoscope that eye doctors still use today, Bates demonstrated that the eye makes continual and minuscule accommodations in order to see. This finding explains why people are so often dissatisfied with eyeglasses. Eyeglasses are intended to "correct" eyesight so that the people wearing them can see an eye chart in a darkened room. However, very few life situations come close to the simulation of the exam room conditions. Many people find their glasses too strong to use in bright light, for example. In turn, some people feel dizzy when they wear glasses. This is because the glasses work best when we stare straight ahead, at stationery objects, and keep absolutely still.

The second radical statement Bates made is that "defective sight can get better as well as worse." In other words, persons who are near-sighted (who have myopia) and far-sighted (who have hyperopia), as well as those who have other conditions, can improve their vision. People may come to a point at which they do not need their glasses, or they may find that they only need their glasses under certain conditions. One of the ways this improvement happens is that people work to strengthen the muscles involved in sight; the other way is by working to re-train the eyes so they see more effectively.

With respect to Bates' third tenet, if you have age-related macular degeneration (ARMD), you know very well that poor sight and disease are intimately related. However, if you are among the many people who had myopia for many years before developing ARMD, I bet you've never thought of near-sightedness as a disease. Yet we now know that all these conditions—myopia, hyperopia, presbyopia, astigmatism, lazy eyes, and crossed eyes—reveal fundamental weakness in affected eyes. We also know that these conditions can be reversed to a great extent through vision training, as well as through the other techniques Bates recommended.

Finally, when looking at Bates' last tenet—the idea that eyesight and overall health are intimately related—we realize his idea reinforces everything I have been saying in this book so far: heal yourself, and you will heal your eyes.

THE DIFFERENCE BETWEEN EYESIGHT AND VISION

Bates translated his complex theories into practical exercises. These exercises are very easy to do and they will work whether you know the theories behind them or not. However, I think it's really important to explain one theory before we go over exercises for vision training. This is the theory that eyesight and vision are different things entirely. Eyesight is a measurement that results from the vision testing procedure. No doubt you are familiar with such testing and most likely know what your eyesight measures in each eye. Now, if we took two people who had the same level of eyesight and put them through a series of *vision* tests, I am willing to bet that their vision would not be at the same level. Instead, I am confident their "seeing" abilities, or their "vision," would differ significantly. This is because vision is a result of much more than the mechanics of the eye. Vision includes memory, experience, and emotions. It is also a function of how relaxed you are at any one time and how accepting you are of what you see.

Bates' approach to vision included exploring the roles all of these factors play. His approach is the basis for the vision training techniques that are widely available today. I want to emphasize how empowering you may find understanding the difference between "eyesight" and "vision." You may have had an experience that many of my patients have also had. They do their eye exercises faithfully and discover that they can see much better. When they come back to me for a traditional eye exam, I tell them that their eyesight is the same. That means that they are still reading up to the same line in the eye chart. However, I fully believe it when they tell me that they can see better, or that their vision is better; now, I understand that there is a lot more to seeing than meets the eye!

Aldous Huxley Meets Dr. Bates

You may be surprised to learn that one of the great writers and philosophers of the twentieth century, Aldous Huxley, benefited enormously from the eye treatment method I will be describing in this chapter. Mr. Huxley's eye problems began with an acute infection that left him blind for eighteen months: after that, he had greatly limited vision, and even that began to fail in his later years. In a state of desperation, he began to work with a Bates vision-training specialist. After several months' work, Mr. Huxley was reading without glasses and had improved his vision substantially. His eye problems, which were of twenty-five years duration, were improving.

Full of gratitude for his own experience, he wrote *The Art of Seeing* in 1942 (now out of print, but available through online bookstores and at many libraries), which relates the Bates Method of visual education to modern psychology and critical philosophy. The following quotation from Huxley's preface gives an idea of how he saw this work in the context of standard medical practice of his day, over fifty years ago.

> *Why, it may be asked, have ophthalmologists failed to make these applications of universally accepted principles? The answer is clear. Ever since ophthalmology became a science, its practitioners have been obsessively preoccupied with only one aspect of the total, complex process of seeing—the physiological. They have paid attention exclusively to eyes, not at all to the mind[,] which makes use of the eyes to see with. I have been treated by men of the highest eminence in their profession, but never once did they so much as faintly hint that there might be a mental side to vision, or that there might be wrong ways of using the eyes and mind as well as right ways, unnatural and abnormal modes of visual functioning as well as natural and normal ones.*

In the following sections, I describe some simple and highly enjoyable techniques for stabilizing and improving your vision. These are adapted from techniques originally outlined by Bates.

EYE RELAXATION AND FOCUSING EXERCISES

Do all the following exercises without wearing your glasses, contact lenses, or sunglasses, and make sure you are in good light. (Your glasses or lenses prevent your eyes from reaching their capacity by bringing things to them.) The purpose of the techniques described below is enhancing your eyes' ability to see. At first, you may feel anxious without your glasses, especially if you are in the habit of wearing them all the time. Before you begin these exercises, make sure that you feel safe and secure. Make sure you are not required to do anything like drive, cook, or take care of a young child while you are doing your vision training techniques. Following these guidelines will help reduce your anxiety. Now, let's review some of the well-known Bates techniques and look at the best way to apply them.

Palming

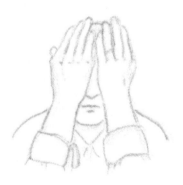

This technique's purpose is to provide the eyes with total rest. After you have done palming for a while, you will improve in your ability to recognize eyestrain. People with impaired sight strain their eyes when they attempt to see more clearly. Palming allows you to develop a relaxed sense around your eyes. Then, you can proceed with the other exercises more smoothly.

To begin palming, sit at a table with your eyes closed. Rub your hands together briefly. Then, rest your elbows on the table and position your slightly "cupped" hands over your closed eyes. Do not exert pressure on the bones of the eye orbit or cheekbones. It's important to support the elbows; that way, the back is comfortably straight and there is no undue pressure on the neck, shoulders, or arms. Be aware, also, of how you position your feet; this is an important part of achieving a relaxed and comfortable posture.

Do not touch your eyes with your hands. Make sure your hands only touch the bony area around the eye sockets. Make sure all light is sealed out, and remain in this position for some time. In this way, you will begin to recognize what it feels like to have relaxed eyes. Do this exercise at least twice a day, working up to fifteen minutes each time. It is worth experimenting very carefully to find the best position for sitting while you are palming, as a very small difference in the support height can have a big effect on your comfort. It can be especially beneficial when your eyes are tired while doing a lot of close work.

Swinging

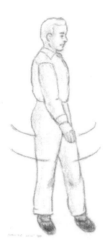 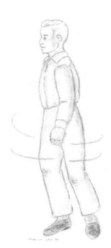

The "long standing swing" is arguably the most important single technique of the Bates Method. This exercise teaches overall relaxation and helps break the weaker eye's habit of staring fixedly at a point. Swinging produces the illusion that objects are moving. Repeated exposure to this phenomenon of apparent movement will encourage a sense of free mobility and improved vision in patients.

To begin this exercise, stand with your feet shoulder-width apart. (Make sure you are wearing comfortable, supportive shoes). Allow your arms to hang naturally at your sides. In one movement, turn your upper body from the waist, so that you are facing one side. You should be making a ninety-degree turn of the body. Keep your head and neck aligned with your shoulders. Keep your eyes looking straight ahead at all times. Immediately twist back to your starting position, and then, in one movement, turn the other direction. As you swing, shift your weight from one foot to the other. The movement should not be greater than ninety degrees from your straight-ahead position, and it may be less if the full movement causes you discomfort. This exercise can be done once or twice a day.

Sunning

Sunning is an exercise that is very soothing and easy to do. It is best done out of doors on a sunny day, but it can also be done outside on a cloudy day or even inside while looking out a window. Sunning helps to rebuild the retina while also improving someone's psychological and emotional state. It also accustoms the eye to light and reduces photosensitivity.

You should perform sunning by sitting in the sunlight, facing the sun, with firmly closed eyes. It is probably best to do this exercise in the early morning, as the sun is rising, or in the evening, when the sun is setting. You should avoid the hours between 11:00 a.m. and 2:00 p.m. when the sun is at its brightest. Slowly turn your head from side to side, while continuing to face the sun. As you turn your head, you will see the image of the sun move across your closed eyelids.

Sunning should be approached gently at first. Build up to a comfortable level until you are performing this exercise twice daily for ten minutes at a time. Sunning should always be followed by a brief period of palming. It is possible that at some point sunning will produce vivid "after-images" in your eyes. This is not a problem. The images can provide a strong focus for your attention and be very relaxing. Still, if these images appear, you should continue palming until they have entirely disappeared and your field of vision has returned to normal. Bates was right! Sunning can help protect the eye against damage and improve the vision in macular degneration. I will discuss this in Chapter 7.

Slow and Rapid Blinking

Slow and rapid blinking is a simple way to quickly relax your eyes anywhere at any time. It increases the production of tears, which deliver nutrients and moisture to the eye. For good sight, you need both nutrients and moisture. To begin this exercise, try relaxing by focusing on your breath. Blink freely and often, but alter your blinking rate. Alternate between fast and slow blinking. Occasionally squeeze your eyes shut for a few seconds: this allows them to rest and shift focus.

"Squeeze blinking" helps you produce tears whenever you need to lubricate your eyes; this also bathes your eyes in nutrients. Squeeze your eyes shut for the count of three. Then, open your eyes wide. Relax your eyes and blink a few times. This is an exercise that can be done many times through out the day to help improve your vision.

Acupressure

Acupressure is a way to increase energy flow to the inner eye. You perform it by applying light pressure and finger massage to certain points around the periphery of the eye. Acupressure can be done before or after palming, and you will find these acupressure exercises soothing and pleasant to perform. While there are many variations to this approach, I am going to make it simple for you to learn and remember, in the hope that you will do this often.

Close your eyes gently and make certain that you do not squeeze your eyes. First, use your thumbs to massage the points at the inner corners of your eyes. Be sure your hands are clean and your nails short.

Second, place your thumbs at the outer corners of your eyes and use the sides of your index fingers to lightly massage the area along your eyebrows.

Third, using the pads of your index fingers or thumbs, gently press along the lower half-circle of bones under your eyes. Move from the outer corner to the inner, using a motion that continues that described in the second step. The tissue in this area is very delicate, so avoid stretching it during this routine. Continue to massage around your eye in ever-widening concentric circles until you have reached your whole face and neck.

What to Expect

I hope your eye exercises and relaxation will feel so good that you will continue to do them without an expectation of specific results. Most of my patients tell me that once they begin these techniques, they feel so great they have little trouble sticking to a regimen. Practicing these exercises is a form of training, done in a relaxed state, which has a "payoff" under stressful conditions. In terms of vision, stressful conditions can include times of emotional tension and attempts to see things beyond one's range of vision. After working on these exercises for some time, you may find that reading simply becomes easier. Often, patients tell me that after practicing these exercises, when they are reading, they become relaxed and see better. However, when they realize they are doing something that used to be difficult for them, they may then "freeze up" because of the awareness. Then, the letters blur again. If this happens to you, use that time to practice the palming and blinking exercises. Many people report they have flashes of extra clear vision at random times. These little "gifts" show you your eyes' capacity to respond to vision therapy. Above all, do not be discouraged if you feel that you are seeing better, but your eye doctor tells you during an eye exam there has been no improvement. Trust yourself!

THE EYEPORT

Microcurrent stimulation, which is described in detail in Chapter 8, can help to improve visual acuity, but after using it, many patients still have problems with functional vision. I remember one patient who achieved excellent improvement in his acuity through microcurrent stimulation. He had over three lines' worth of improvement on the eye chart, and his eye doctor could not believe the results. When I spoke to the patient, though, he told me he was still having trouble reading and seeing street signs.

I realized that although he had good acuity, he still lacked good function. So, we gave him specific exercises—spatial exercises—so he could become more aware of his peripheral vision and develop skills to translate his new vision into function. There are many aids that can be used in vision therapy for this purpose, but I believe a very good introductory device is the Eyeport.

My friend, Dr. Jacob Liberman, developed this device over a thirty-year period. Dr. Liberman noted that many patients had poor visual function regardless of their acuity. He developed a device that improves visual function called the Eyeport. As a side benefit, in some cases it actually improves acuity, too. This device does three things. First, it balances the autonomic nervous system by using color. Red is sympathetic, while blue is parasympathetic, and the center signifies balance. (I describe how this works in more detail in the following paragraphs.) Second, it also helps balance the left and right sides of your body. Most people do not have harmony between the left and right sides of their body, and this can result in lower visual function. The Eyeport helps balance this disharmony—and, third, it also helps you find your vision's sweet spot.

The Eyeport looks like a space age radar gun. It uses a series of alternating blue and red lights. If you recall, we talked about the autonomic nervous system in Chapter 3, and it has two components—the sympathetic and the parasympathetic. The sympathic component is related to the color red. Red increases energy and shifts the autonomic system to the sympathetic side. The parasympathetic component is related to the color blue. Blue has a relaxing or slowing affect on the autonomic system. The lights on the Eyeport alternate red and blue. When the red light goes on, the Eyeport stimulates the sympathetic system; when the blue light goes on, the Eyeport stimulates the parasympathetic system. So, by using the Eyeport, you stimulate both ends of the autonomic nervous system: red, blue, red, blue. This bouncing back and forth between colors pushes the autonomic nervous system to the center or to its balance point.

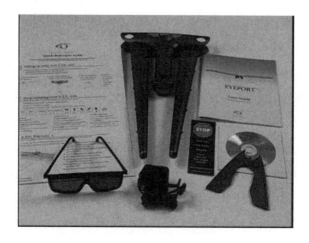

The Eyeport system can be purchased
from Dr. Lieberman at www.exercisetheeyes.com for about $250.

To use the Eyeport, you wear special glasses that have one red lens and one blue lens. You wear these while looking at the Eyeport's red and blue lights. Suppose you have the red lens in front of your right eye and the blue lens in front of your left eye while you are looking at the lights. When the red light goes on, you will only see the color blue using your left eye. Your brain tells you that you are seeing blue with both eyes, but really the red lens in the right eye is canceling out the image of the red light. When the blue light goes on, the situation is reversed. This visual technique coordinates the left and right side of your body. This is important because you need equal visual perception in both your eyes to have good visual function. Most people have an imbalance between their eyes, which results in disequilibrium. When you develop an eye disease, usually it starts on one side or the other. Overall, this therapy helps balance the left and the right side of the body through pleasant and easy exercise.

The third thing the Eyeport does is help you find your vision's sweet spot. What is your vision's sweet spot? It is the spot on your retina where you have the sharpest vision. Let me explain in more detail. Many people who have eye problems can read the eye chart, but they struggle to do so. They read very slowly, turning their heads, moving their bodies side to side, reading the letters in a faltering or halting way, and even guessing. They may say, "F, no, G," pause, and then say, "B, no, F." They eventually read the letters correctly, but the whole time, they are trying to find their vision's sweet spot (although they probably don't know they're doing so). They can pick out individual letters, but there are disconnections between their functioning retinas, their brains, and their bodies. If you know where that sweet spot is, it is very easy to read. Of course, with a healthy macula, the sweet spot is easy to find, too. However, if you have a scar or blind spot, it becomes more difficult to find that retinal sweet spot. The Eyeport helps you find the sweet spot, so that you are able to use what you've got. The FDA has approved the Eyeport system as a method for improving functioning vision. The Eyeport is widely used by children to help with dyslexia, learning disabilities, and attention deficit disorders.

Vision therapy is easy and can be done at home. The Eyeport machine comes with instructions on paper and on DVD to make its use really clear. In only twenty minutes a day, you can improve your visual functions dramatically. I recommend you do the exercises every day for twelve weeks. Once you begin to do these vision exercises, you will begin to notice that you are functioning differently in space. You will realize you are reading better. You are then using your eyes properly instead of improperly, and you will develop good, positive skills that will help your visual system continue to improve.

For example, even though I have 20/20 vision, I still went through this program. The program helped me with reading. I am an impulsive reader. When I read, I like to jump ahead; I just don't stay focused on the material as it is printed. After a course of vision therapy, I found I had become a better reader.

If you have kids or grandkids who are having problems at school, vision therapy is something that can really help them. It will aid the neurological system, as well as the eye's ability to read, track, and function properly. One of the biggest problems I see with kids is that their visual systems are not being developed. Those of you who are my age will remember that when we were kids, after school we would go outside, run in the woods, play baseball, and do a lot of physical activities. Today, when kids come home, they turn on the TV or computer. They just focus on a small area of a screen; they are not developing their peripheral vision or their hand-eye coordination. The visual system is not incorporated with the motor system, which causes severe developmental problems.

How can these problems be addressed? We have a lot of fun ways to do so. We do a great deal of vision exercises and motor activities with the children we treat. For example, one vision exercise involves the use of the trampoline. (This incorporates the benefits of jumping on a trampoline discussed in an earlier chapter.) For this exercise, we write the alphabet on a blackboard and place the blackboard near the trampoline. As the kids jump up and down on the trampoline, we ask them to read every other letter. Then we ask them to read every third letter, and then we ask them to read every third letter backwards. All the while, they are going up and down on the trampoline. Then, we ask them to cover one eye, then the other eye. Then, we ask them to jump up and down while alternating feet. It is amazing how such a fun exercise also quickly develops their visual systems.

Many of these techniques can be applied to other learning skills. I am learning how to play the piano in a traditional way: I am taking piano lessons. My piano teacher uses skills that are similar to the ones we use in vision therapy. She continually changes the environment in small increments, so that she challenges me. Say, for example, that when I am home practicing I can play a musical piece perfectly well. My teacher will put the metronome on, change the rhythm a little bit, and tell me not to look at the piano keys. Then, she will tell me to play it. Alternatively, she might put some background music on, or start talking to me while I am playing. We create these types of environmental changes in our vision therapy, too, in order to place stress the muscular system. That way, true learning occurs.

VOSTAR TEST

Another thing we use in vision therapy is a special test, the VOSTAR, which measures a patient's perception in space. This test is necessary because many of us feel that we perceive our environment properly when, actually, we do not. For example, suppose I look at a glass on a table. My mind tells me the glass is in a certain place on the table. However, let's say that my visual system is not aligned properly and so the glass is actually two inches to the left of where I perceive it to be. I reach for it and miss the mark. Then, I make a subconscious adjustment, so the next time I reach for it I am more accurate. Over time, I learn to move my hand just a little bit to one side so I can reach my target.

This is just like using a handgun with a very poor sighting mechanism. If you are always hitting the target on the left, you learn to adjust the gun to the right so you can hit the target.

When we do these visual perception tests, it is really amazing to see how many people have misaligned visual perception. This misalignment causes stress in their visual systems and contributes to a decrease in their function. In vision therapy treatment, we work on special exercises that help your eyes develop much better alignment. These exercises help you realign your visual system, so you can function better in space.

Much of the time, structural problems with the body, including the way you stand and your head tilt, are due to the alignment of your visual system. Exercises that straighten your eye muscles can straighten your whole body's configuration. As we get older, our bodies tend to stoop, we tend to look down, and we don't look up. Our upward gaze becomes restricted simply because we are not using it.

Dr. O.A. Da Silva, a professor of ophthalmology in Portugal, has done research on a new syndrome, Postural Deficiency Syndrome, which may affect over 10 percent of the population. This condition consists of postural problems that can lead to painful head and neck conditions, dizziness, balance disorders, anxiety, concentration difficulties, and learning disorders. He believes that ocular misalignment can cause major structural and functional problems in the body. I attended one of his workshops, where I saw case after case of people who had difficulties that had been diagnosed as neurological diseases, vertigo, and so on. Dr. Da Silva's approach dramatically changed these people's abilities to function, instantly, just by giving them specialized prism glasses. Prism glasses shift the image you see, helping the eyes to shift in a proper alignment. One way to think about how this works is to imagine what happens to your car when its tires are out of line. The car will shake and will not stay in a straight line. After the tires are aligned, the car's function will improve.

I have one amazing case to tell you about. My patient, an elderly woman who could not walk without her walker, was very dizzy and weak. She always needed help getting up out of chairs. She had many of the characteristics of Postural Deficiency Syndrome. I took some measurements of her eyes to try and correct this misalignment, and then, based on those measurements, asked her to wear a pair of specialized prism glasses. Suddenly, she was able to get up from her chair without assistance and even walk without assistance!

Remember, in vision therapy we look at far more than just acuity; we observe how your body functions so we can work on the whole idea of functional vision and the things we can do to improve it. This philosophy has become a big part of my practice. It is a big part of helping our patients both to regain their acuity and their ability to function in space.

Here's an interesting fact to consider: About 80 percent of the neurological system is tied into the eyes. Think about all the cranial nerves that are related to the eyes; there are six of them. The facial nerve makes seven. In total, there are twelve cranial nerves, and seven of them—over half—are related to the eyes. As a result, people with many types of neurological problems can really benefit by improving their vision. For example, patients with Parkinson's disease have a certain Parkinsonian gait and posture. However, if they use prism glasses, they can change their posture. I have seen a lot of Parkinson's patients walk better due to this treatment.

One group of optometrists, the College of Optometrists in Vision Development (www.covd.org), is really keen on alternative therapy, particularly alternative vision therapy. This group's website invites you to search for a trained optometrist in your area. The group has done a great deal of exciting work that actually shows neurological damage can be reversed. For the longest time, people believed that once someone injured neurological tissue, that tissue could not be regenerated. Recent studies show, in contrast, that neurological tissue can actually be regenerated if it is stimulated.

I have had a long-standing interest in vision therapies and eye exercises because I believe that they can help regenerate damaged eye tissues. A typical eye doctor will say that once you start suffering from macular degeneration or glaucoma damage, the problems cannot be reversed and tissue cannot be regenerated. However, I believe you can experience a great deal of improvement by taking a multi-disciplinary approach, look at your lifestyle basics, add homeopathic remedies to stimulate your body, and then introduce some type of vision therapy to your routine.

NIDEK MP-1

The Nidek MP-1 is another recently developed, exciting piece of technology that can aid vision. The Nidek MP-1 is an auditory feedback machine that helps retrain the eye to utilize the retinal sweet spot. When people have macular degeneration, they have scar tissue right in the center of their eyes. So, when they try to read, they try to force that damaged area to do the reading. Likewise, when they look at an object, that blind spot (or scar tissue) is right in the center of their eyes as they look. The brain can't tell the eye to move over a little bit and read outside that scarred area. I hear about this all the time from patients: "Dr. Kondrot," they say, "if I could just move that blind spot to the side, maybe put it over here, I would be fine. But every time I look straight ahead, it's right in front of me!"

Using this machine, the Nidek MP-1, we can actually measure what the best area of the retina would be for becoming the new center of vision. Our goal is to get the brain not to focus on the scar tissue but, instead, to use a point of vision along the scar tissue as the focus. In the Nidek MP-1, we have a device that measures retina sensitivity in different areas, and thereby finds the best new, central vision location (or area of fixation). Then, once that point has been located, this machine retrains the eye to use a different part of the retina as the central fixation area through an auditory feedback system.

Perhaps sometimes this can work too well. One of our patients, who struggled with reading because of his macular degeneration, went through a series of treatments to retrain his eyes. He went from struggling to speed-reading after just a few sessions. Soon after, we were alarmed when he called us up from his Porsche. He said, "I am doing hairpin turns here in Colorado at eighty miles an hour. I got my depth perception back!" This is a true story. So now we have to have you sign waivers and release forms in case you become overexcited about your new vision capabilities.

A recent study published in *Applied Psychological Biofeedback* (Volume 34, 2009) shows that the Nidek-MP can improve acuity, reading ability, and fixation in patients with macular degeneration. The study reveals how ten treatments of ten minutes each had powerful results, as shown in the following measurements made on the treated patients:

- 300 percent acuity improvement
- Improvement in reading speed (an average of twenty-eight words per minute)
- Better fixation and focusing

VISION THERAPY IMPROVES VISUAL FUNCTION IN MACULAR DISEASE

A recent article in the *Archives of Ophthalmology* (from the May 2008 issue) reports on some of the benefits of vision therapy. In the study, researchers randomly assigned 126 patients with low vision (related to diseases of the macula) to one of two groups. The first group joined a vision therapy program, which consisted of weekly face-to-face sessions with a visual therapist and daily homework assignments (in which patients learned techniques to improve visual function). The other group joined a waitlist and received no vision therapy.

After four months, the group that received vision therapy had a significant improvement in all aspects of visual function, including reading ability. In the group that did not undergo visual therapy, vision and functional ability declined. This study's results show that vision therapy can benefit patients with macular degeneration.

Another interesting study, conducted in a Virginia hospital, focused on forty patients with macular degeneration; each of them did only vision therapy. The patients did not receive homeopathy, vitamins, or minerals, etc. After a ten-week program, using only vision therapy throughout, the majority of the macular degeneration patients had measured improvements in acuity, reading speed and comprehension, and tracking and fixation. This shows vision therapy can be a big part of rehabilitating your eyes if you have an eye disease.

SHOULD YOU DO IT YOURSELF
OR FIND A PROFESSIONAL?

In this chapter, I have described ways to improve your acuity, but also ways of taking that acuity and making it improve your functional vision. Because you have a certain level of vision, by improving your whole visual and sensory system, whatever level of vision you have will work better for you. In the Bates Method section, I provided a number of vision exercises that are deceptively simple, yet very powerful. Anyone, anywhere, with any level of resources and with any visual level, can work on these exercises and experience profound results.

Want to work with a professional? Find a well-trained vision therapy eye doctor in your area by searching on www.covd.org. Think of vision therapy for help with learning disorders, macular dysfunction, macular degeneration, glaucoma, or vision loss. It can also aid people with traumatic brain injuries, because vision therapy helps redevelop neurological and visual systems.

Perhaps your experience has been the same as the writer Aldous Huxley's. Up until now, maybe no one has suggested that there might be a better way to use your eyes. Welcome to a brave new world!

CHAPTER FIVE NOTES

Books

Huxley, Aldous. *The Art of Seeing.* New York: Harper & Brothers, 1942.

Mansfield, Peter. *The Bates Method.* London: Vermilion Press, 1992.

Quackenbush, Thomas R. *Relearning to See: Improve Your Eyesight Naturally!* North Atlantic Books, 2000, Berkeley, California.

Schneider, Meir. *Self-Healing: My Life and Vision.* New York: Viking Penguin, 1987.

Organizations

The American Vision Institute – Vision Training Resources
1111 Howe Street
Sacramento CA 95825
(916) 929-8831
www.visiontherapy.net

The Bates Teachers Association
www.seeing.org/index.html

College of Vision Development
www.covd.org

Homeopathy

My favorite approach to treating any disease is using homeopathy. Surprisingly, many people don't know what homeopathy is. They confuse it with herbal therapy or with vitamin programs. Those methods are important, but they are not homeopathy. Homeopathy is a specific science: It is a specific branch of medicine based on certain laws of healing. One reason I love homeopathy is that its practitioners still use the same textbooks people used 250 years ago. Those textbooks have not changed. When I went to medical school, half of what I learned there was outdated by the time I was a senior. Modern medicine is not based on laws; it is based on current theories, and those theories change. In fact, they change every couple of years. Overall, however, a general idea links these theories. Practitioners of conventional modern medicine look outside the body. They believe certain organisms or accidents cause disease, and if they can take care of the external factor(s), the patient will get better.

Homeopathy has a consistent theory that makes a great deal of sense to me. In contrast to conventional medical practitioners, homeopathy practitioners do not look outside of the body for solutions. They believe that disease comes from the inside of the body, and if people change their insides, their outsides will change. The primary law of homeopathy is the "law of similars." This law states that a substance that causes a symptom or disease in a healthy person will cure the same symptoms or disease in a sick person. For example, if someone has a high fever, we could give him or her a homeopathic remedy—a substance that causes high fever in a healthy person—and he or she would then recover from the high fever.

HOMEOPATHIC RESEARCH

Practitioners have researched all the substances used in homeopathy in order to determine their effects. Many people think that homeopathy is not based on science, because the typical design of pharmaceutical drug research, which they recognize as scientific, is different from what practitioners to prove the effectiveness of homeopathic remedies. Actually, however, homeopathic "provings" (homeopathic research designs) are far more scientific than any pharmaceutical research practices. For one thing, in the early stages of testing, pharmaceutical drug research is done primarily on animals, and research focuses on only one physiological effect. In contrast, in homeopathy, when practitioners do a proving, they (myself included) have no preconceived idea about what they will find. They look at what symptoms arise after the substance or remedy is taken.

How is a proving done? A group of healthy individuals all take some small white pills (the most common form of delivery for homeopathic remedies) for a period of time, usually about a month. During that time, they do not know what is in those pills. They record all the symptoms—physical, mental, and emotional—that arise in them. Then, they meet and share their experiences with the person(s) conducting the research. The measurement of the symptoms induced in the greatest number of individuals indicates the symptoms that the remedy will cure in sick people.

For instance, let's say that most of the people who took one remedy during a proving noticed a throbbing headache; perhaps they noticed some light sensitivity, maybe they got a fever, or maybe they felt an unusual amount of anxiety. We can conclude that the homeopathic substance that caused these symptoms will also cure them. So, later on, when a patient's symptoms include a throbbing headache, light sensitivity, and anxiety, along with an elevated temperature, a homeopathic practitioner knows that if the patient receives that remedy—because it matches that disease state—he or she is likely to recover, and to recover quickly at that.

Homeopathic practitioners do not only look at physiological symptoms; we also look at mental and emotional symptoms. In other words, we look at an entire picture of a person. Homeopathy encourages the belief that a person has one abnormal vibration or one state of disharmony, which produces many different symptoms. The belief in homeopathy is there is one abnormality, regardless of the number and/or types of symptoms he or she exhibits, so only one homeopathic remedy is required to restore him or her to health. You do not need a remedy for your headache, another one for your eye problems, another one for your digestion, and so on. People who follow that form of homeopathic practice are not able to tap into the real powers of homeopathy. The individuals who make these kinds of recommendations are practicing homeopathy in the conventional medicine manner, in which there is a drug for each type of symptom. If you seek conventional medical assistance for your symptoms, you will receive a drug for each symptom. Your gastroenterologist will give you medication for your stomach; your eye doctor will give you eye drops; your allergist will give you allergy medication. Each person will give you medication or treat part of the problem. Conventional medical doctors do not address the entire disease state or, rather, the whole person.

THE LAW OF SIMILARS

One of the most important laws in homeopathy is the law of similars, which I have already mentioned briefly.

Let's look more closely at this law and see why it is so important to understanding disease and the proper ways to treat disease. In homeopathy, if you have a headache, we practitioners prescribe a medicine that causes a headache; if you have a fever, we prescribe something that causes a fever; if you have diarrhea, we prescribe a medicine that causes diarrhea. You might be thinking, "Well, Doctor, I don't want that medicine! I've already got diarrhea; I don't want something to make it worse." However, this approach actually helps treat the disease: it does not make the disease worse. In fact, in order to achieve true health, it is essential to treat symptoms this way.

In homeopathy, we understand that the body has a certain kind of wisdom, and believe there is a single reason why a person develops a particular set of symptoms. Homeopathy's assumption is that the body wants to be in balance, or to achieve "homeostasis." Yet things like shock, trauma, or grief can put the body out of balance. At that point, the body reacts by developing physical symptoms. A homeopathic practitioner then prescribes a medicine that supports the body's attempt to restore health.

When you are out of balance, your body (and mind and emotions, too) reacts a certain way: It produces symptoms, and these new symptoms are what is necessary to help your body regain and maintain homeostasis. By taking a substance that supports the body's reaction and attempts to achieve homeostasis, you help your body regain health quickly—very quickly. Conventional Western medicine, also called allopathic medicine, does not support this belief. Instead, this medicine treats patients by using opposites. If you see a conventional practitioner because you have diarrhea, you will be given a medicine that causes constipation; if you have a fever, you will be given a medicine that lowers your temperature. The end result of treating with opposites is very detrimental to health because diseases are pushed deeper into the body and become increasingly severe.

DIRECTION OF HEALING

If a child has a problem with eczema, he probably goes to a pediatrician, who puts him on steroid cream. The eczema goes away, and the parents are happy. But what happens later on? Eventually, the child develops asthma. Then, his asthma is treated with drugs that suppress the symptoms. Everything goes along well until, eventually, the patient "suddenly" develops arthritis or cancer because traditional medicine drove the original disease deeply into his body. In contrast, when that same child receives homeopathic treatment for his asthma, he finds that the asthma gets better. Then, guess what happens? The eczema comes back. The body heals in a certain way: Old symptoms often arise again so the homeopathic remedy can cure them, too.

Another law of homeopathy is that disease tends to go from the outside to the inside, and when you heal the person, the healing goes from the inside to the outside. When I went to homeopathic school, I learned that if you give a patient a good homeopathic remedy and he or she develops a rash, that's a reason to celebrate. Of course, many times, when this happens, the patient is not happy and will need to be counseled in order to avoid further "suppression" (pushing the disease back into the body). In this case, if a patient steps away from homeopathy and uses steroids or cortisone to treat the rash, he or she is suppressing the body's healing action and actually pushing the disease deeper into the body. Conventional doctors don't look at the timeline of the disease; they don't look at how the disease may have changed from one form to another. They don't try to understand how the body has suppressed disease. Most of you reading this book have probably lived a life of suppression episode after suppression episode.

When people get pneumonia, they take antibiotics to suppress the fever; if they have arthritis, they get steroid shots and the swelling goes away. For example, suppose a patient has arthritis, which begins with just an ache in the left knee. The patient goes to the doctor. The doctor says nothing is wrong and may suggest that the patient take some aspirin, or something like that. Then, when the patient gets some more swelling, it can be treated it with an injection or surgically drained; then the patient gets scar tissue. If you take that same patient, who by that point has severe arthritis and a scarred leg, and you treat him or her homeopathically, guess what is going to happen? The inflammation may come back. The leg may swell, again. Then, however, the swelling will go away, and in a short time the patient will be healed. This demonstrates another law of healing: healing occurs in reverse order of symptom appearance.

One thing I have observed, in my years of practicing medicine and homeopathy, is that the process of suppression occurs with every disease that has received improper treatment—even eye diseases. For example, let's look at cataracts. A cataract is a superficial problem, much like a skin problem, that begins to blur a person's vision. In fact, this similarity is because the skin and the eye are related; the human eye lens is derived from the neuroectoderm, the primitive embryological layer that also produces human skin. If you see a traditional practitioner for this problem, the eye doctor will tell you that having cataracts is an easy problem to fix. A simple operation will correct this and give you perfect vision. However, nothing is done to investigate what caused the cataract or to look at the underlying problem. Homeopathic laws are ignored! Patients listen to their eye doctors and they have cataract surgery to improve their vision, which works for a time. However, guess what happens years later? They may develop macular degeneration or another problem later on.

Even ophthalmology literature states that, according to the facts, incidents of macular degeneration increase after cataract surgery. People in the eye care profession state that this increase occurs because the patients are getting older. Macular degeneration would have occurred in them anyway, even without the cataract surgery. However, I believe this increase occurs because of suppression. Cataract surgery does not treat the real cause of the disease. I don't want you to think that I am totally against cataract surgery, because in many cases cataract surgery is necessary for improving vision. I am against the absence of homeopathic treatment. When a person receives homeopathic treatment, his or her body is going to be much stronger.

I look at homeopathic treatment as a catalyst (or as the catalysts) that simulates the body to heal. This healing is something magical. I have experienced its magic in the healing of my own body, and that has made me very enthusiastic about using it for my patients. Years ago, when I was a busy ophthalmic surgeon, I trained for triathlons; I was very active. Then I developed severe asthma, which really limited my life. I could not exercise anymore, and I took a lot of traditional medications. I even took steroids. These medications caused a tremor in my hands, and you can't be a very good eye surgeon if you have a hand tremor. So, I took a beta-blocking drug to reduce my tremor, but this drug made my asthma worse. That was my life. (Many of my patients have had the same type of experience, even though they may have other conditions.) After a certain point, the drug cycle just does not work.

My neighbor happened to be the city's top pulmonary doctor. I went over to his place one day and said, "Dave, I want my old lungs back. Where are my old lungs? What can I do to get my old lungs back?"

He said to me, "There is no cure for adult-onset asthma; just be happy the medication is helping you." He also made the comment that unfortunately, not only is there no cure for asthma, but that I would probably die from it. Prior to this exchange, I thought my neighbor was my friend.

At this time I was using homeopathy for aches and pains, and it was working miraculously. I wondered if it could help my asthma, too. To find out, I went to a professional homeopathic who talked with me about my symptoms and prescribed a remedy. Nothing happened. At that time, I thought homeopathy worked on the basis of the placebo effect (that if you believe in it, it will work). I believed, but nothing happened. However, I persevered. I took a second remedy and had somewhat better results. Then, I took a third remedy, and that completely cured my asthma.

HOMEOPATHY FOR EYE DISEASE

At that point, I realized that if homeopathy could work for a chronic disease like asthma, maybe it could work for eye problems, too. I did some research and was amazed to discover that in the early 1900s, a large percentage of eye doctors were homeopathic practitioners. New York Island Hospital used to be a homeopathic eye hospital; homeopathic eye doctors had their own society; and these doctors published a scholarly journal. I began to immerse myself in studying homeopathic treatments for eye disease, and I was astonished at what I uncovered. I decided to incorporate what I learned about homeopathy into my practice. In order to become proficient in homeopathy, I enrolled in a professional training program for homeopaths and studied there for four years.

My studies gave me new ways to treat patients. I'd like to tell the story of one of the first patients I treated homeopathically. This patient, who had glaucoma, was an engineer. He fit the stereotype of an engineer in appearance: white shirt, very narrow tie, pocket protector, notebook, and NASA haircut. He came into the office with a notebook full of his records of his eye pressure levels, the time of the day when he took his eye drops, when he ate, and so forth. He kept all these parameters on a graph and was trying to understand how different events correlated to his eye pressure. Meanwhile, he was losing his vision, and the eye drops were not controlling his pressure. At that point, surgery was the only option. However, since I was studying homeopathy, I thought it might be helpful in reducing his pressure and stopping some of his medications. He was interested in trying this. I gave him a remedy that I believed suited his personality and temperament, as well as his symptoms, and asked to see him in a couple of months to measure the remedy's effect.

I had been seeing this patient for at least four or five years. He came in every visit looking the same. He was always wearing a white shirt, narrow tie, and pocket protector, and carrying his notebook. Nothing about him ever changed. However, when he came into the office for his follow-up visit, after the homeopathic treatment, the office staff members said, "Dr. Kondrot, Mr. Smith is here, but we did not even recognize him."

When I walked into the examination room and greeted him, I saw the change right away. He was wearing a sweater and a leather coat. His hair was a little bit longer. No pocket protector was in evidence, and no notebook either. I asked him if he had noticed any changes since taking the homeopathic remedy.

He said, "No, not a darn thing. It did not do a thing for me."

I told him I had noticed that he was dressed differently.

He said, "Yeah, I changed my style a little bit—you know, got away from the engineer look."

When I measured his pressure, it was much lower. As a result, we were able to reduce his medication—we did not completely eliminate his medication, but we reduced it. This example reveals what homeopathy does; it provides a profound shift, not just in your body, but also in your whole personality. That's what always amazes me.

I have another story that supports this point. One of my two pet cats developed a severe eye infection. His eye was filled with pus. It was horrible. I was treating him with a homeopathic remedy and getting no results. I thought I would have to take him to the vet, and expected to be ridiculed. "Oh, so you are the great homeopathic eye doctor! I can see you've really helped your cat. So, now you come to me," the vet said in my imagination. Then I recalled that

I knew a brilliant homeopathic vet, Susan Beal, who has a practice in Pennsylvania. I called Susan and asked for her help in finding the correct homeopathic remedy for my cat.

Susan started by taking a homeopathic case. She asked questions such as, "What does the cat do in the litter box? Which corner does the cat go to, and how much time does it spend there? How does the cat eat, and where does it like to sleep?" She asked questions about his personality and what his fur looked like too, before prescribing the remedy. Three days after the cat took the remedy Susan recommended, it had a normal eye! I could not believe it. Even though I have a strong faith in homeopathy, I sometimes think it may not work in a certain case (such as my cat's). I thought this was a miracle.

Another of the amazing experiences I have had with homeopathy occurred with a patient who was himself a doctor. This doctor, who was lecturing in Pennsylvania while I still practiced there, developed a sudden onset of blindness after a central retinal artery occlusion (a stroke to the eye). In the ophthalmology training program I attended, I learned that this is a very serious condition; if it is not treated in the first five minutes after it occurs, there is no hope for recovery. I saw the doctor five days after the occlusion, and he was totally blind in that eye. The only treatment he received was placement on blood thinners, in order to prevent it in his good eye.

This doctor grew up in India, where homeopathy is very popular. He wanted me to suggest a remedy and treat him homeopathically. I told him immediately that I had not ever treated a condition like this with homeopathy, and I really did not know if homeopathy could help him. However, I believed that a good remedy would produce a possible change in his body and that might help his vision. I took his homeopathic case in order to learn about his nature and personality so I could prescribe the correct remedy. (Remember, in homeopathy, our goal is to treat the person and not the disease. Two people with the same disease will most likely need two different remedies). After learning about him, I gave him the homeopathic remedy that best matched his symptoms and personality. I told him to take the remedy twice a day and give me a call in a couple of days. If he felt no effect, I would consider changing the remedy.

I lost track of time. A week went by, and I still had not heard from him, so I called him. I was astonished when he told me that on the second day of taking the remedy, he had begun to get some vision back. Several days later, his vision was perfect. (He also told me that he had visited a retinal specialist who told him, based on the total recovery of vision, that the original diagnosis must have been incorrect.)

These miracles occur in homeopathy because you treat the person, not the disease. People often ask me what I took to cure my asthma. It does not matter what I took; what I took may not work for you. You will need to take something else in order to cure *your* asthma—or, rather, to cure *you* of your asthma. This is why you need to see a well-trained homeopath. The practice of homeopathy is a very complex art and science. It offers over 3,000 remedies, and you need to take the correct one *for you* to get results. A good homeopath can help you achieve this, and this book's resource section can help you find a homeopath in your area.

IN HOMEOPATHY, LESS IS MORE

One major reason why traditional medical practitioners do not accept homeopathy is because homeopathic remedies are given in dilute substances, or micro-doses. Homeopaths usually dilute a substance beyond its physical presence. What happens is the following: If you dilute something by a hundred, only one hundredth of the substance will be present. If you dilute it again by a hundred, only one ten-thousandth will be left. If you continue to dilute it, a point will be reached when there is no longer any substance left. Conventionally trained doctors cannot understand how this can be effective; therefore, they don't accept it. However, scholars have conducted and published research that proves water has a memory and can retain the imprint of a substance, even after successive dilutions to a point in which the physical substance no longer exists. In 1988, one researcher, Jacques Benveniste, published a study called *Human Basophil Degranulation Triggered by Very Dilute Antiserum Against IgE* in the journal *Nature*. In this study, which was duplicated at six major European universities, Benveniste used extreme dilutions of anti-IgE, dilutions beyond the presence of any physical substance, and created a solution that still showed biological activity. Transmission of biological information could be related to the water's molecular organization. Information of a chemical substance is imprinted or left on water molecules. The water molecule continues to carry this imprint of information to continue to show biological activity.

In the following section I describe a case in which my patient had extraordinary results using homeopathic treatment. Perhaps this will motivate you to find a homeopath and be treated homeopathically yourself.

A Woman on Guard Against Further Macular Degeneration

Elizabeth, a seventy-six-year-old healthcare agency owner, had a look of suffering on her face when she walked into my office. "I'm worried," she began. "What is going to happen to me?" She had a vascular form of macular degeneration and was very anxious to get her vision back. She'd seen many specialists and had been through more than ten laser treatments, but still wanted better results. A recent hypertensive crisis, in which her blood pressure had spiked to 220/146, hadn't helped matters.

Elizabeth described herself as a skeptical person. In order to make informed decisions about her treatment options, she wanted a great deal of information. She also suffered from considerable anxiety. During her childhood, someone had robbed her home; the thief had come up through a trap door. After the event, she and her sister had taken turns staying up at night. Elizabeth still carried fear based on that traumatic event. "I frequently fear that someone is in the room when I'm home," Elizabeth told me. "I sleep with the lights on all night long; I lie on my left side facing the door; and I have a small, loaded gun ready. I'm on my guard. I suppose I could solve this problem if I had a dog. Then the dog would be on guard instead of me." Typically, each night she would sleep for a couple of hours and then wake up between two and three in the morning. Her fears worsened when she was alone. When her husband was in the hospital, for example, she stayed up all night.

Elizabeth also preferred to read books about simple, small-town life—books in which neighbors visit with and look out for each other—in order to escape. She liked the feel of soft clothes and desired creature comforts.

My eye exam revealed that she had cataracts and ARMD (age-related macular degeneration) in both eyes. In the right eye, she had central scarring, because of the laser treatments; in the left macula, she had retinal pigmentary changes and large drusen (accumulation of toxic waste). She had 20/400 vision in her right eye and 20/40 in her left eye. In addition, she had hypertension and anxiety.

As I studied her case, the remedy *Calcarea carbonica* seemed strongly indicated. The type of person who needs this remedy often has issues about security in the home and enjoys the simple pleasures of life. Before prescribing it, though, I also needed to consider the remedy called

Arsenicum album, because it often helps people who have many fears, especially fears about their health or of robbers. Both remedies can also be used for patients who have cardiovascular complaints. After deliberating, I selected a *Calcarea arsenicosa* remedy because it covered both of my patient's *Calcarea* and *Arsenicum* aspects.

I started Elizabeth on a dose of high-strength, gentle-acting *Calcarea arsenicosa*. She took the remedy for six months. While I usually see my patients every three months, Elizabeth did not return to see me for a year. When she returned, she reported she had initially waited two months before starting the remedy, because she was afraid it might make her feel worse. However, once she started taking the remedy, she began feeling better. Her energy improved, so she felt more industrious at her business. She could relax more easily, and she felt happier. Her fear of being robbed had disappeared, and she didn't feel as fearful at night. To top it all off, when she returned, I noticed her vision had improved by two lines on the eye chart.

While this remedy was extremely effective for Elizabeth, please do not run out and buy it if you have eye disease and fears. The chances that the exact same remedy will work for you are very slim. Instead, find a homeopath to treat you. Homeopaths have years of training in observation and inquiry so they will be able to find the right remedies for individual patients. Suppose I see one hundred patients with cases of macular degeneration. It is possible that each person will need a different homeopathic remedy. This individualized concept is one of the major reasons that conventional doctors misunderstand homeopathy. They are accustomed to prescribing the same drug to all patients who have the same disease.

Glaucoma

The homeopathic approach to treating glaucoma is very different than the conventional approach, which uses eye drops, laser treatments, and surgery to lower glaucoma patients' pressure. In fact, the standard medical method of lowering pressure by blocking aqueous production is similar to treating someone's high blood pressure with medication that stops blood production. It does not make sense! The same is true of conventional methods that use injections to treat macular degeneration. While they might help reduce the swelling, these injections do not address the degeneration's underlying cause.

Based on the law of similars, or the idea that the substance that causes a disease will cure it, we can take this homeopathic approach to treating glaucoma. Let's look at substances that produce an adverse change in the eye pathology similar to that found in glaucoma, such as substances that cause eye pressure elevation or substances that cause the optic nerve atrophy or damage. Several substances have been shown to be effective at lowering elevated eye pressure. Significantly, there is just not one substance that lowers this pressure. As homeopaths, we look at the whole person and at all of his or her symptoms, whether they are mental, emotional, or physical. So, perhaps one hundred people who all have glaucoma might each need a different homeopathic remedy.

The approach that fits my interest in treating glaucoma is finding remedies that are effective at reversing or stopping optic nerve damage. A good example of the homeopathic approach to treating optic nerve damage can be found in reviewing a condition called "toxic amblyopia." Toxic amblyopia is a toxic reaction in the orbital portion (or the papillomacular bundle) of the optic nerve, caused by various toxic and nutritional factors. Toxic amblyopia is usually bilateral and symmetric (which makes it similar to glaucoma damage). Alcoholics with toxic amblyopia may have developed the condition due to the underlying cause of malnutrition. Other substances that can damage the optic nerve include tobacco, lead, methanol, chloramphenicol, digoxin, ethambutol, DDT, aniline dyes, and many other chemicals (including several over-the-counter and prescription drugs). Many of these substances have been proven and prepared as homeopathic remedies, and most of them are listed in homeopathic literature as being effective in glaucoma treatment.

Homeopathy can be extremely helpful in the treatment of glaucoma. Please remember, however, that glaucoma can be a very serious disease. Typically, if I am treating a patient homeopathically, I do not allow the patient to stop taking glaucoma medication until I observe the proper homeopathic medication is having a pressure-lowering effect.

Even then, I will gradually monitor the patient's pressure while tapering the glaucoma drops.

Cataracts

How can homeopathy be used to treat cataracts? The government of India's Central Council for Research in Homeopathy, which is part of the Ministry of Health and Family Welfare, has stated that a tincture of *Cineraria maritima succus*, made from the dusty miller plant, is the drug of choice for preventing the development of cataracts. The recommended therapy is one to two drops in the eye, three to six times daily. William Boericke, a prolific homeopathic writer, describes the tincture as being most effective in traumatic cases and states patients should receive one drop four or five times a day for several days. John Henry Clarke, MD, who also wrote extensively about homeopathy, adds that patients should simultaneously receive specific homeopathic treatment internally.

The best-reviewed article on cataract treatment is *The Homeopathic Treatment of Incipient Senile Cataract, with Tabulated Results of One Hundred Cases*, written by A. B. Norton, MD, and published in 1891 in the *North American Journal of Homeopathy*. This retrospective study looked at the results of homeopathic cataract treatment in 295 patients. One hundred of these patients underwent treatment for longer then three months. The results showed improvement in 58 percent of the cases and no change in 42 percent, The best indication of success for participants in this group was their level of vision before treatment;

those in earlier stages of cataract problems had the most improvement. So, the earlier you treat cataracts, the better the results.

Case Study: A Ballroom Dancer with Advanced Cataracts

"I love to ballroom dance," lamented a seventy-eight-year-old patient of mine. "I even reached the silver level [in ballroom dancing], but now, because of my poor vision and dizzy spells, I can no longer compete." Sylvia, a real estate broker, felt depressed, hopeless, and withdrawn about her situation. Since her last eye exam, when she had been told she had macular degeneration and cataracts, she had noticed that her vision was worsening and reading was becoming difficult. She lived in fear of occasional spells of vertigo, which would come on suddenly and cause her to fall down like a rock. The room would seem to spin from left to right, and she'd be left debilitated and "quivering like an old lady." She would be so weak that her arms and legs would shake. Twice, this happened when waking up from bed, and she could only pull herself up with great effort.

She feared these dizzy spells would return when she encountered stress. "If I'm having a stressful conversation, I feel that my balance will leave me," Sylvia added. "It's as if the bottom is dropping out of my stomach, and I become light-headed." The ringing in her ears, which was associated with her vertigo, was also annoying.

As I took her case study, Sylvia added that she was not in a relationship and that her sexual drive had never been very high. However, she noted, "There is a lot of sexuality in dancing. I especially like all the provocative aspects of Latin dancing."

After a thorough eye exam, I diagnosed her with macular degeneration (myopic degeneration with atrophic changes in the retina), advanced cataracts in both eyes, and poor vision (20/300 in the right eye and 20/700 in the left eye). None of this was good news for an active woman.

However, in Sylvia's case, homeopathy provided an avenue for addressing such a complex set of symptoms. I thought the *Sepia* remedy was a strong contender. A.B. Norton's recommendation of *Sepia* as the number one remedy to consider for women with advanced cataracts also supported this prescription. In addition, women who need *Sepia* can feel much better when they exercise, and they often love to dance.

For Sylvia, I prescribed *Sepia* at a gentle but high strength, to be taken as needed. *Sylvia* took the remedy for six months. At her follow-up appointment, eight months later, she reported that she could now read a menu, which was something she hadn't been able to do for quite some time. She had experienced a 70 percent improvement in her vision. She could see street signs more clearly and colors more vividly. An eye exam showed that the vision in both her eyes had improved; she had improved from 20/300 in the right and 20/700 in the left to 20/200 in both eyes. As an added bonus, the dizziness and ringing in her ears were gone.

From Self-Care to Professional Care

Homeopathy is medicine for the people. It should not be obscured under some academic guise. I believe everybody should assemble a personal or family homeopathic first aid kit and begin to use it at home. Through my practice, I have met mothers who have young kids. When they begin to use homeopathy at home, they cut down pediatric visits and continue to improve the health of their children. When I treat a person with homeopathy, I ask entirely different questions than a "regular" eye doctor does. I'm trying to find out the following: What is the patient's body trying to do? What might be this condition's underlying cause? Before me, I see a *person with* an eye problem, not just an eye disease. Then, once I have looked at the underlying causes—once I have evaluated what is going on with the patient physiologically, mentally, energetically, and emotionally—I can select a good homeopathic remedy that will not just take care of the eye problem but also take care of the whole person. If I am able to take care of the whole person, then the patient and I can both look forward to him or her regaining health in a really dramatic manner.

It is important that a person trained in eye disease as well as homeopathy treats serious injuries to, diseases of, and chronic conditions of the eye or of vision. If that sort of person is not available in your area, you should seek out the combined efforts of an eye care professional and a qualified homeopath.

So, how do you find a good homeopath? The Council for Homeopathic Certification (www.homeopathicdirectory.com) maintains a list, organized by state, of approved homeopaths. These are practitioners whose education meets certain standards and who have become certified in homeopathy after passing rigorous testing. They use the designation "CCH" after their name. Another source, the American Institute of Homeopathy, is a trade association of medical and osteopathic physicians, dentists, advanced practice nurses, and physician assistants. On the association's website (http://homeopathyusa.org/home.html), you can search for well-qualified, licensed professionals who also practice homeopathy. A related organization, the American Board of Homeopathic Therapeutics, grants physicians and osteopathic physicians a title, designated by "DHt," to indicate that they have the prerequisites for homeopathic practice and have successfully passed both a written and an oral examination.

Homeopathy is not a licensed practice in most of the United States. Some homeopaths, such as myself, may be licensed in another profession, such as medicine, nursing, or chiropractics, and also practice homeopathy. Other homeopaths, called "professional homeopaths," only practice homeopathy. When selecting a homeopathic practitioner, the important thing to ask about is his or her training: did he or she attend a full three- or four-year program to learn homeopathy?

HOMEOPATHIC MEDICINE AS FIRST AID

In addition to treating the more serious, chronic eye conditions discussed in this book, homeopathy can also treat injuries and acute conditions as a type of first aid. Homeopathic first aid can work for both you and your family members. Even if you are taking a prescription drug for your eyes (or for any other condition, for that matter), you can still use and benefit from these highly effective, natural treatments.

Because of my commitment to encouraging people to use homeopathy in first aid and home care, I have developed a list of remedies (widely available at health-food stores, drugstore chains, and even at some grocery stores) that can be used as first aid for common eye problems. These remedies are all in pill form and should be taken orally, even though the problem is in the eye. The easiest way to purchase these remedies is to look for a display of "blue tubes" manufactured by Boiron Laboratory in the stores. The tubes will be lined up in alphabetical order. The following picture illustrates how the display looks in most stores:

The remedies themselves are in small blue tubes, each about the size of a lipstick, and are quite inexpensive, around $7 each. Each tube has enough pills for several doses of the remedy. To take the pills, turn the tube upside down and rotate the clear cap until several small white pills fall into the cap. Each dose is about three to five pills: the precise number is not important. Once the pills are in the cap, pop them into your mouth and let them dissolve. Be sure you have not eaten, brushed your teeth, chewed gum, or anything like that for at least fifteen minutes before taking the pills. After taking them, wait fifteen more minutes before putting anything else in your mouth.

In the next sections, we will discuss which remedy to take for which condition. While homeopathic remedies have Latin names, you will find that homeopaths use standard terms. Thus, even though the remedies' names may seem strange to you, they will be used consistently in every source. If you decide to go shopping for remedies, take this book or a list with you. If you really get excited about homeopathy, you can even buy a first aid kit (available from many sources), and consult one of the books listed at the end of the chapter in order to become more skilled at treating yourself and your family (that includes your pets, too).

HOMEOPATHIC REMEDIES FOR THE EYE

Over the years, I've found the following six remedies to be extremely useful for treating acute conditions that affect the eye. Significantly, they are all members of the plant kingdom, a fact that corresponds to the theory that "sensitivity" is a key feature in the symptom profiles of patients who benefit from homeopathic remedies made from plant sources.

Belladonna: Sudden Onset

Belladonna is a well-known acute remedy and a first-line homeopathic treatment for any sudden inflammatory reaction. I have often used it on patients with cases of pink eye (epidemic keratoconjunctivitis). A patient may have classic *Belladonna* symptoms, such as a rapid onset of redness with marked swelling, extreme photophobia (light sensitivity), or irritability. *Belladonna* can reduce these symptoms quickly and resolve the infection faster than any antibiotic can. Other symptoms that may indicate *Belladonna* treatment for any acute eye problem are a glistening appearance of the eye, dilated pupils, or a wild expression in the eye.

Another acute problem that I have successfully treated with *Belladonna* is central retinal vein occlusion. This occurs when arteriosclerotic thickening or arterial spasms cause a sudden blockage of blood flow in the veins of the eye. (In the eye, the small veins and arteries share common sheaths at the points where they cross each other.) Ophthalmologists call this problem "blood and thunder retina," a phrase that describes the rapid and substantial accumulation of blood inside the eye. The result, for the patient, is sudden vision loss, along with marked inflammation and redness in the retina. Of course, a case of sudden onset with marked redness and swelling is a classic indication for *Belladonna* treatment. *Belladonna* can stop the retinal hemorrhage, help soak up the blood in the eye, and improve the patient's vision. In contrast, in traditional ophthalmology the only treatment for this condition is laser surgery. While surgery stops bleeding, it destroys healthy retinal tissue and often further reduces the vision.

Aconite: "Arnica of the Eye"

Aconite napellus, another commonly used acute remedy for the eye, is often called the "*Arnica* of the eye" because of its all-purpose use for treating eye trauma (*Arnica*, in turn, is an all-purpose homeopathic remedy for treating general trauma). *Aconite* often helps patients when they develop conjunctivitis after exposure to cold, dry wind.

Aconite has other uses, too. It is also the number one remedy to consider for treating sunlight-based photophobia. I have found that solar keratitis responds very well to *Aconite*, too. In this latter condition, a patient's cornea becomes inflamed after it is exposed to sunlight reflected from snow, sand, or water. Aconite is also a very valuable remedy for treating pain experienced after undergoing laser surgery (for example, laser surgery might have been prescribed to treat nearsightedness). The laser used for these surgeries is an ultraviolet laser, which has part of the sunlight spectrum.

Staphysagria: Not Just for Styes

Patients who need *Staphysagria* often develop styes, which are infections of the glands at the eyelash base. A sty can also be viewed as a beautiful representation of the classic nature of *Staphysagria* because it is an enclosed, purulent pocket hidden by normal-looking skin. Likewise, a person who needs *Staphysagria* will often show off a sweet exterior, while holding anger and indignation inside, which eventually leads to pathology. A sty takes a very long time to develop before finally releasing its toxins; similarly, a person who needs *Staphysagria* typically holds onto anger and indignation for long periods of time. Thus, I use this remedy as my first line of treatment for styes, especially if the patient in the case has a history of indignation.

I have also observed some cases in which patients who have deep eye pathologies, such as glaucoma and macular degeneration, respond well to *Staphysagria*. Recently, a patient came to me with a loss of vision in her left eye due to inflammation of the optic nerve (known as "optic neuritis"). Upon taking her case, I learned that her problem developed after she had an argument with her daughter. The daughter's boyfriend did not want my patient to see the couple's child, her granddaughter. This event caused her great psychological stress and indignation. She had also had some dental work around this time. Interestingly, the *Staphysagria* symptom profile includes "ailments from indignation" and "ailments from dental work/surgery." My patient had suffered a double whammy. I treated her with *Staphysagria*, and her vision returned to nearly normal after several weeks. She was also able to deal with her anger towards her daughter. Normally, if vision returns after a bout of optic neuritis, it does so slowly, over three to six months. The remarkable and rapid improvement of this patient's vision (as well as her mental state) can be attributed to the rapid action of *Staphysagria*.

Pulsatilla: Infections and More

Pulsatilla is another homeopathic remedy commonly used to treat eye infections, especially bacterial infections that produce a yellow-green discharge. *Pulsatilla* treatment can also assist with many other eye pathologies. Remember, one important characteristic modality of this remedy is that a person with related systems will feel worse in warmth and better in the cold; in addition, the person will feel better when he or she goes outdoors.

Several years ago, I treated a woman suffering from a retinal hemorrhage. She had a marked loss of vision. She wept when telling me about her symptoms and indicated she had very strong, fixed religious ideas. Both of these characteristics are strong indications for *Pulsatilla*. She had a marked preference for cool air and a craving for creamy comfort foods. I prescribed *Pulsatilla*, which quickly resolved the hemorrhage and improved her emotional stability. Her vision also improved, which, most likely, would not have occurred without homeopathic treatment.

Hypericum: Soothes Pain

Hypericum, a well-known remedy for treating injuries to nerve-rich tissues, is a favorite remedy of mine for corneal injuries. Compared to other parts of the body, the superficial cornea has the highest concentration of pain nerve fibers. Anyone who has experienced a small scratch to the cornea will agree that corneal injuries are tremendously painful. Consider taking *Hypericum* for any corneal injury, such as a scratch to the eye, a problem that arose from wearing contact lenses too long, or a surgical procedure that injured the cornea.

Euphrasia: Heals Eye Irritations

Euphrasia officinalis, made from the plant commonly known as "eyebright," is my first and best remedy for external irritation of the eye. Symptoms that this treatment is required can include redness, irritation, and feeling like sand is in the eye. Allergic reactions, dry eyes, and infections can all respond well to Euphrasia. The key indicator for *Euphrasia* treatment is an acrid eye discharge. (In contrast, the need for the remedy *Allium cepa*, which is made from the red onion plant, includes the symptom of non-acrid eye discharges that occur simultaneously with acrid nasal discharges.) I often suggest to patients with this condition that they drink herbal eyebright tea and use the tea as an eye compress. Unfortunately, the herbal tincture is becoming more difficult to obtain in the United States (although some sources still exist). Because *Euphrasia* is a semi-parasitic plant, the USDA has banned the importation of *Euphrasia* seeds for fear it will take over other plants.

How to Choose a Remedy

As you can see, some remedies can be used for the same condition. For example, *Aconite, Belladonna,* and *Hypericum* can all be used to treat injuries. The best way to approach choosing a remedy is to have several remedies on hand. Try one and if the first one does not work well after about fifteen minutes or so, then try another. See the next section for guidance on changing remedies and repeating doses.

How Often Should You Repeat the Remedy?

The biggest mistake people make when taking homeopathic remedies is to repeat the remedy choices too often. This is not bad for people, nor is it toxic, but it can make the medicine less effective over time. My colleague and editor, Gloria St. John, has devised a helpful visual aid, the "Injury and Acute Condition Dosing Chart," that people can refer to so they know how often to repeat remedies when taking them for acute conditions or injuries. This flow chart also offers people guidance on when to try a second remedy. Please consult this chart, included below, for guidance in treating yourself with homeopathic remedies effectively.

HOMEOPATHIC INJURY AND ACUTE CONDITION DOSING CHART

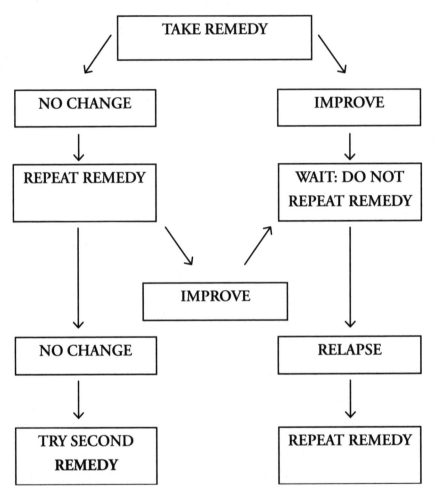

GOLD HILLS HOMEOPATHY

Gloria St. John, Homeopath
Sacramento and Ione, California
www.goldhillshomeopathy.com
info@goldhillshomeopathy.com
© Gloria St. John, 2007

After you have read this chapter, I hope you will feel motivated to purchase some homeopathic remedies or maybe buy some books on the subject to help you treat minor injuries and illnesses with homeopathy at home. That way, you avoid drugs and doctor visits that are unnecessary. I have provided a rich list of resources at the end of the book that you can use to get yourself started. Most importantly, after reading the chapter, I hope you will consider adding homeopathic treatment to any other treatment you are receiving for your eye conditions.

CHAPTER SIX NOTES

Homeopathic Resources and Directories of Homeopaths

American Institute of Homeopathy
www.homeopathyusa.org/

Council of Homeopathic Certification
www.homeopathicdirectory.com/

National Center of Homeopathy
www.homeopathic.org/

Where to Buy Homeopathic Books

Homeopathic Educational Services
www.homeopathic.com/

Minimum Price Books
www.minimum.com/

Where to Buy Homeopathic Remedies

Hahnemann Laboratory
www.hahnemannlabs.com/

Natural Health Supply
www.a2zhomeopathy.com/

Washington Pharmacy
www.homeopathyworks.com/

Sleep and Light Therapy

N ow that you are eating well and drinking plenty of water, you've become familiar with homeopathy, and your autonomic nervous system is well balanced, the next step in the healing process is to be sure that you sleep well. People often underestimate the importance of sleep, and of sleeping in complete darkness. We know that our seasons have a cyclical rhythm. Shorter days and longer nights signal winter. Longer days and shorter nights signal summer. This rhythm provides other signals for birds to migrate, bears to hibernate, leaves to change, and so forth. Under normal circumstances, these changes also bring a shift in the days' dark-to-light ratio. Not any more. Now, days are not necessarily bright and nights are not dark. This change upsets our important, and natural, biological rhythm.

This change affects the pineal gland, located deep within the brain. The pineal gland's process is directly dependent on the circadian rhythm of night and day. During daylight, the pineal gland produces serotonin, an important neurotransmitter (a chemical that relays messages between nerve cells). It also accumulates melatonin, a natural hormone that regulates sleep. At night, the pineal gland stops producing serotonin and instead makes, and secretes, melatonin. The release of melatonin helps trigger sleep and helps you stay asleep.

Dr. Abraham Haim, a biology professor at the University of Haifa, has studied the adverse effects of light at night (LAN) extensively. He conducts his ongoing research at the Israeli Research Center for the Collaboration of Photochronobiology, and he has published numerous papers on LAN-related subjects. In some of his studies, he points out that lit-up cities and light at night are relatively new phenomena in human existence; we have only had artificial light at night for about 130 years. Dr. Haim has demonstrated correlations between LAN and the following health problems: cancer (especially of the breast and prostate glands), obesity, and macular degeneration. Macular degeneration increases with LAN, especially if the light is in the blue spectrum. (Most commercial indoor lighting and all external lighting are in the short, blue wavelength range.)

The problem is that light at night gives an improper signal to the pineal gland. The result is it does not produce melatonin. The body needs melatonin, not just for good sleep and to balance circadian rhythms, but because melatonin is also a very powerful antioxidant. This means that melatonin scavenges for free radicals, the cells that contribute to chronic disease and cancer. This interesting fact shows how nature protects the human body. In the winter, when we are exposed to harsher elements as well as to other people's germs, the long nights encourage our bodies to produce more melatonin naturally. If we disrupt this natural pattern and stay awake while using artificial light, we are compromising our own immunity.

HOW BAD IS LIGHT AT NIGHT (LAN)?

Increased light exposure at night causes a decrease in melatonin production and an increase in abnormal cortisol at night. Cortisol is an important hormone; it is secreted by the adrenal glands and is involved in the regulation of a number of metabolic functions. Under normal conditions, it should be at the highest level in the morning, and very low at night.

If you look at a satellite map of the earth at night you observe areas with a very high density of light. These areas are usually concentrated in large metropolitan areas. One research group looked at these geographic areas with high-density lights and compared them with maps of breast cancer. There was a very high correlation of occurrences of breast cancer in the areas of the world that have high light concentration at night. You first thought might be that the increase incidence of cancer has nothing to do with light but perhaps the pollution and stress of living in a metropolitan area. The researches used lung cancer as a control. Lung cancer is associated with high levels of pollution. Surprisingly there was no correlation with lung cancer. Light at night, it was then concluded, was responsible for this increase in cancer. Not surprisingly, occurrences of prostate cancer also correlate to LAN countries. In addition to cancer, other health conditions, episodes, and systems are adversely affected by light at night. These include heart attacks, the immune system, obesity, and, of course, macular degeneration.

Light at night is harmful to both people and animals, studies show. Researchers have conducted several interesting studies on animals that showed that light exposure at night adversely affected the animals' reproductive systems and their ability to adapt to cold temperatures (also at night). In fact, many of the animals exposed to light and then to cold died due to their inability to adapt to the new conditions. In another study, mice were injected with human breast cancer cells and subjected to varying degrees of light interference at night. The study's outcome showed the mice that developed the largest tumors also had the most interference or exposure to light at night. Those receiving melatonin at night had lower tumor growth; the mice that had eight hours of daylight and sixteen hours of darkness had the lowest amounts of tumors.

Scholars conducted similar research to test prostate cancer development in mice exposed to light at night, and the results were nearly identical. Overall, results showed that the presence of melatonin protects against both breast and prostate cancer development in mice, even when the mice were exposed to light at night.

Other studies performed on rats examined the effects of light wavelengths on tumor size. Blue illumination produced a much greater tumor volume; blue light blocks the production of melatonin. Red illumination had very little affect on tumor volume, presumably because red light does not block melatonin secretion.

Melatonin and Heart Attacks

Heart attacks occur more frequently in the early morning due to an increase in the clotting of blood. One study examined the connections between Prothombin time (or clotting time) and light exposure, especially LAN exposure. The study found that patients who experienced long days with light interruption had a much lower PT or Prothombin Time, which increased the risk of clotting.

The Effects of LAN on the Immune System

In one study, conducted on mice, researchers found more frequent occurrences of atypical lymphocytes (white blood cells in the immune system) when the subjects only received a short amount of light during the day and encountered light interference at night. Mice exposed to a short day that had no light interference at night and received melatonin at night had fewer atypical lymphocytes.

In addition, shorter days and light exposure at night correlate to increased occurrences of the flu in the winter and general weakness in many people's immune systems.

Obesity and Insufficient Melatonin

Studies performed on rats have also documented increased occurrences of obesity when subjects experience light exposure at night. This finding is not so surprising, since melatonin is a hormone and we understand that much of obesity is caused by disruptions in the hormone system, particularly disruptions connected to hormones secreted by the adrenals or insulin secreted by the pancreas.

Blue Light at Night Decreases Melatonin Secretion

Mercury in light bulbs shifts the bulbs' wavelengths toward the blue spectrum. This is especially true of new LED (long emitting diode) lights and CFLs (compact fluorescent light). The blue light produces more stimulation of non-photoreceptor cells (these regulate melatonin) than photoreceptor cells (these do not regulate melatonin). LED and florescent lights also increase pollution, due to the toxic components within them that must be disposed of when they break. While these light bulbs might be more economical, this shift toward blue light they provide is potentially extremely harmful for your health and vision.

Formerly, people only used fluorescent lights in offices, stores, and places of business. However, now, because the bulbs use less energy, people are starting to use them in their homes. One problem with fluorescent light, in addition to it not being a full-spectrum light, is that it has a wavelength of about 428. (Any light source with mercury tends to have a wavelength of 428, which is in the blue spectrum, but it is a harmful type of blue.)

Numerous research articles have been published, their findings indicating that early degeneration in the eye produces a substance called "lipofusion," which is one of the components of the drusen (waste products accumulated in the retina) found in age-related macular degeneration. Apparently, the lipofusion absorbs light in the spectrum of about 428 nanometers, thereby causing further damage to the eye. Anyone who has early macular degeneration, or is experiencing early degenerative changes to the eye, is extremely sensitive to the wavelength of light generated both by fluorescent light bulbs and all the new, high-energy light bulbs that contain mercury. These bulbs are disastrous, and they are going to increase occurrences of macular degeneration and eye diseases. They are also bio-hazardous. If you break one, you have to be very careful when cleaning it up and disposing of the shards.

Because of this sensitivity to this wavelength that some eye patients have, many eye doctors recommend something called a "blue blocker." Blue blockers are lenses with a yellowish tint that block the harmful blue wavelengths of light and help preserve the health of your eyes.

However, one question I get frequently from patients is "But, Dr. Kondrot, don't you recommend using blue light as a treatment for my eyes?"

My answer is yes; I do recommend it. However, the blue light used in your light treatment is of a different wavelength and intensity than the harmful blue light you receive from mercury lamps at home and work. Receiving blue light in any form during the night suppresses melatonin production. Do your light therapy during the day when blue light is helpful for your body. *Minimize all light exposure at night.* When the sun sets, it is time to turn off the lights and go to bed! Try making this a habit and see what happens to your vision and health.

Light and Macular Degeneration

Studies support a relationship between decreasing melatonin levels and macular degeneration. In fact, some researchers propose that the melatonin decrease experienced by the elderly may be an important factor in ARMD initiation. In one study, one hundred patients who had ARMD received three milligrams of melatonin every night for a minimum of three months. The researchers followed fifty-five patients as they observed the protocol for more than six months. After six months of treatment, the study's findings reveal, the patients' visual acuity had generally been kept stable. The majority of patients had a reduced pathology in regard to macular changes. Thus, these findings help us conclude that the daily use of three milligrams of melatonin seems to protect the retina and to delay the progress of macular degeneration. (No significant side effects were observed during the study. Resetting the Pineal Clock, Volume 1057, published December 2005 Ann. N.Y. Acad. Sci. 1057: 384–392 (2005) by CHANG XIAN YI.)

SLEEP AND DARKNESS: IMPORTANT CONCLUSIONS

Turn off all the lights in your home at night. In particular, please strive for total darkness in your bedroom at night. Purchase and install light-blocking window coverings; do not keep a nightlight at your bedside; and remove the television and alarm clock (if light-based) from your room. The smallest amount of light that hits your skin can suppress your pineal gland's melatonin secretion. For further protection, consider taking three milligrams of slow-release melatonin at night and strive to get adequate sun exposure during the day.

Melatonin Supplementation

In China, researchers conducted an interesting study on melatonin supplementation. During the study, over two hundred people who had macular degeneration disease took a melatonin pill at night and slept in totally dark rooms. At the study's conclusion, a large percentage of subjects experienced a dramatic improvement in their vision; some even achieved complete resolution of the advanced wet form of macular degeneration. People achieved these results just by sleeping well in a dark room and supplementing with melatonin over a specific period of time.

Although there is no agreement among clinicians about the correct dosage of melatonin to take or even about its value, melatonin is still available as a supplement. Two forms of melatonin supplementation are available:

the natural form, which comes from animals' pineal glands, and the synthetic form, which is made from certain chemical compounds. While natural melatonin may pose a risk to humans because it can be contaminated with animal viruses, synthetic melatonin is safer to use because it is free from biological contaminants.

Each night, the pineal gland produces about two to twenty-five micrograms of melatonin. The amount varies depending on a person's age, the degree of darkness in the sleeping environment, and the length of sleep. Melatonin is related to the pigment melanin, which is essential for the integrity of the eye. One cellular layer of the eye is even called the "pigment epithelium" because it is so heavily pigmented. Some of the earlier changes we see in macular degeneration are related to pigmentation, including the loss of pigment, pigment clumping, pigment dysfunction, and the accumulation of drusen in this area of the eye. The above study shows that getting a good night's sleep, in darkness, helps the body produce a hormone that in turn produces pigment that is essential for good vision.

Complete Darkness

The whole idea of sleeping through the night in total darkness is interesting. The researchers of the above study believed that any light coming into the room whatsoever would suppress the pineal gland to some extent. They determined the room must be completely dark. Some people think if they have a sleep mask on, or if their heads are under the blanket, they are in a dark room. However, if their hands are outside of the covers, even the illumination of your alarm clock hitting the skin can suppress pineal gland activity. So, I recommend that you make sure you sleep in a totally dark room, especially if you have an eye problem. If you need to get up during the night to use the bathroom, then I suggest you purchase room motion detectors. You can plug these into ordinary wall sockets. As soon as your feet hit the ground, the motion detector lights will come on and you will be able to find your way. Another option is to keep a flashlight by your bed. The key, though, is to sleep in a totally dark room.

The amount of melatonin produced each night declines as a person ages, which is reported to be the reason why older people have difficulty sleeping. There is another side to this equation, too: You need proper light exposure during the day in order to establish a good circadian rhythm. Circadian rhythms are physical, mental, and behavioral changes that roughly follow a twenty-four-hour cycle. The rhythms primarily respond to environmental light and darkness, and they are found in most living things, including animals, plants, and even tiny microbes. Unfortunately, most of us live in environments where we function under very poor illumination (including using fluorescent lights and dimly-lit rooms) even during the day, and we do not get enough exposure to full-spectrum light in order to make sure that the circadian rhythm in our body is natural and optimal.

Researchers at the University of Rochester conducted a very interesting study on the topic in a nursing home. One of the biggest problems nursing homes have is getting nurses to work at night. The night shift is really tough for nurses because that's when all the problems occur. When seniors are lying in bed at night, they start to get aches and pains and want help from the nurses. Seniors also need to go to the bathroom, and most require assistance to do so. Overall, the residents do not sleep well, which drives the nurses crazy.

The study's investigators observed that, during waking hours, all the people in the nursing home gathered in a dimly-lit room where there was no sunshine. The residents played cards and watched television in poorly illuminated, indoor settings. The investigators decided to expose half the residents to full spectrum light every day for thirty to sixty minutes, late in the afternoon, and leave the other half in the normal light environment. Then, the investigators would observe any changes that took place in the subjects' sleep cycles. Close to 99 percent of the group that had the exposure to the bright light were sleeping at any given time the nurses checked on them during the night, compared to 60 percent of the people from the group that did not have exposure to the bright light.

Next, the investigators did research to see if any other light wavelength would duplicate the full-spectrum light's effects. Only one other wavelength duplicated the full spectrum: 470 nanometers, or the color that is sky blue.

So, the investigators concluded that getting exposure to full spectrum light or to blue sky will help someone's whole circadian rhythm.

This study's findings have amazing implications. We need to expose ourselves to more bright, natural light during the day to keep the circadian rhythms of our bodies functioning. A proper circadian rhythm not only helps us sleep well, but may also reduce the occurrences of cancer and chronic disease.

As a result, one thing we now recommend in our practice is that patients regularly go outdoors and get exposure to sunlight. Currently, exposure to sunlight is once again gaining acceptance in medical literature because people have such extensive vitamin D deficiencies. The best way to strengthen the immune system is by exposure to natural sunlight, which produces vitamin D in the body. We recommend that our patients go out every day, late in the afternoon, and get at least one hour of sunlight exposure in order to help keep their circadian rhythm going and experience better sleep at night.

ULTRAVIOLET LIGHT: A CAUSE OF OR CURE FOR MACULAR DEGENERATION?

Back when I was completing my ophthalmology residency, it was widely accepted among my colleagues that UV light caused cataracts and macular degeneration. This belief was based on one study conducted on animals in which their eyes were continuously exposed to ultraviolet light—in a manner that could not be duplicated in humans. To evaluate it fairly, we must look closely at the study's design, especially at the subjects' continuous, uninterrupted exposure to light, which produced the pathology. These conditions were far from the ordinary conditions experienced by human eyes when encountering sunlight. Of course, the animals developed results, but the researchers' conclusions were false. According to one expert, this evaluation is comparable to someone putting his or her hand in a blast furnace and then stating that heat is bad for our homes. Too much of anything can be hazardous to our health. High levels of oxygen in premature infants cause eye damage. Does this mean that oxygen should be avoided?

Another idea that has been indoctrinated in us, and in our society, is that sun exposure causes cancer, specifically, malignant melanoma. We lather ourselves with suntan lotion and protect our bodies from the sun to minimize our chance of contracting this deadly disease. However, is it true that sun exposure causes melanoma? At least one study, which focused on women in Australia, demonstrated that more of the women who were exposed to fluorescent light at work developed melanomas than those who were continuously outdoors—even those whose favorite pastime was sunbathing.

In his book, *Light: Medicine of the Future*, Dr. Jacob Lieberman reports on the following benefits of UV (sun) light:

- Activates vitamin D synthesis
- Lowers blood pressure
- Increases heart efficiency
- Reduces cholesterol
- Helps in weight loss
- Helpful in psoriasis treatment
- Increases sex hormone levels

Another study showed that retinal pigment epithelial cells would not divide unless they were exposed to low levels of ultraviolet light. What this means is that UV light is necessary for our health in a number of ways! Particularly, severe deprivation of UV light might be contributing to the development of macular degeneration.

While I am not suggesting gazing at the sun as a treatment for or way to prevent macular degeneration, I believe moderate exposure to sunlight can be the best overall medicine for our eyes. My suggestion is that you spend at least one hour a day outdoors and get exposure to sunlight. (If you are very fair-skinned, and it is summertime, you may need to work up to a full hour of exposure or cover up a bit.) When you are outside, take time to remove your sunglasses, eyeglasses, or contact lenses (unless you've had cataract surgery). Do not look directly at the sun. Instead, absorb the sun's reflected light with your eyes. Even on a cloudy day there will be benefits. *Caution! If you have had cataract surgery, you have lost the protective benefit of the human lens. You need to reduce exposure to UV light and protect your eyes with sunglasses.*

Do not use sunscreen during this daily sun exposure. SPF 15 blocks about 95 percent of the beneficial light that produces vitamin D from reaching your skin. That is where vitamin D is made—on the surface of your skin, by your natural oils, when your skin is exposed to sunlight. So, don't be too clean either. If you are constantly bathing you will remove the natural oils on your skin that help in the production of vitamin D. Some studies' findings also suggest that sun exposure to the head actually decreases vitamin D production, because direct exposure to the head somehow depresses the pineal gland's activity. If you want to get sunlight's maximum benefits, then you should wear a hat and mainly expose your body or limbs to the sun, not your face and head. So, you can get naked and go outside, but put on a hat—and maybe dark glasses, so nobody can recognize you!

LIGHT THERAPY: MEDICINE OF THE PAST, HOPE FOR THE FUTURE

The longer I am involved with alternative medicine, the more I appreciate the power of light therapy and the therapeutic effects it can have on balancing the body. This therapeutic effect holds true whether the light therapy is "informal" (meaning that you deliberately balance your light and dark exposure, as recommended in this chapter) or used as a medical treatment. Getting that ultraviolet light into your system can be a very powerful and effective way of improving all chronic diseases. Read on to see how light and color can actually be used in therapeutic settings to heal eye disease and other disorders.

BATES WAS RIGHT!: RESEARCH CONFIRMS SUNNING IS BENEFICIAL

Dr. William Bates, a controversial turn-of-the-century ophthalmologist whom I discussed earlier, believed that stress caused all eye diseases and that people could cure those diseases by relaxing the eyes. He advocated light therapy, in the form of sunning, over a hundred years ago, and that technique just might be a key to the prevention and treatment of macular degeneration. While I described his techniques of palming, swinging, and sunning in Chapter 4, there is actually more to and other forms of "sunning."

Until now, nothing in the field was more controversial than Bates' technique of sunning. Bates believed that the eyes benefited from sunlight and that people could look directly at the sun (with closed eyelids) or at the brightest light without injury or discomfort. Bates cautioned that, just as people should not run a marathon without training, people should not look directly at the sun without training. Bates suggested people expose the white part of the eye, or the sclera, to direct sunlight for a few seconds at a time; he also advocated exposing closed eyelids to direct sun.

In his book, *Perfect Sight without Glasses*, Bates describes a treatment that uses a magnifying glass to focus sunlight on the closed lid of an eye. He advised patients to expose their closed eyes to direct sunlight for at least three minutes a day; on dark days, he advised using an infrared light source for "sunning" indoors. He advised people that sunning could help refractive problems, like nearsightedness and farsightedness, as well as problems like glaucoma, cataracts, and macular degeneration.

During my ophthalmology training, my professors taught me that looking at the sun was bad—that doing so could burn the retina, leading to blindness. In class, we even studied several cases of retinal damage that occurred after sun gazing, including the case of a man who took several doses of LSD and then proceeded to sun gaze for several hours.

Recently, several respected journals have published articles about research that supports Bates' theory that sunlight can be beneficial to eye health. Here, I summarize the research using human subjects; there are interesting studies conducted on animals that you can read about in this book's resources section.

The study "Low Level Laser Therapy Improves Vision in Patients with Age- Related Macular Degeneration," by B.T. Ivandic et al., involved 193 patients with all forms of macular degeneration. An infrared laser (780 nanometers) was used to irradiate a three-millimeter spot on the conjunctiva near the macula of the eye. Each eye received a total of four laser lights lasting forty seconds, twice a week over two weeks. Visual acuity improved for more than 95 percent of the patients, while 86 eyes with wet macular degeneration had reduced bleeding. In addition, metamorphopsia, impairment of color vision, and scotomas decreased.

In another study, called "Early Diagnosis of Ocular Hypertension Using a Low Intensity Laser Irradiation Test," authors B.T. Ivandic, N.N. Hoque, and T.P. Ivandic found that infrared light, when shined on the sclera, significantly reduced intraocular pressure in the majority of patients. A thirty-second treatment reduced intraocular pressure by 50 percent in some patients. Others received less of a reduction, while the remainder had no pressure-lowering effects. The patients with existing glaucoma all had a greater pressure-lowering response, compared to those who did not have glaucoma. According to the authors of the study, this test might help to distinguish which normal tension patients and which patients with slightly elevated pressures might be at risk for developing glaucoma. Low-intensity laser irradiation may be an important tool for treating ocular hypertension and glaucoma.

Caution: It is important that you never conduct any light treatment on your eyes, the eyes of another person, or the eyes of animals. Light treatment must be done by an eye professional. I hope there will not be a long delay in incorporating these methods into routine eye care. A list of the most progressive eye doctors, including many who practice light therapy, can be found at www.covd.com.

Color Therapy and the Treatment of Eye Disease

There is nothing new under the sun. Color therapy sounds like something that belongs to interior design, not in the doctor's office! You may be surprised to learn that there is a long history of using color in eye disease treatment. Dr. Harry Riley Spitler first developed this clinical science, which he called Syntonics (from the word "syntony," which means "to bring into balance") in the 1920s. His research and clinical studies validated the profound effect that light has on human function and health. Since then, a now seventy-three-year-old institution called the College of Syntonics has investigated the effects of color therapy in the treatment of eye disease. Evidence shows that disease is caused by an imbalance in the autonomic nervous system. Stress—yes, we have heard of that word—certainly contributes to this imbalance and to disease; moreover, stress, as we learned in Chapter 3, can also be the fuel that sustains disease and prevents healing.

Researchers believe the mechanism of stress in the body over-stimulates the sympathetic nervous system and suppresses the parasympathetic. When the parasympathetic system is suppressed, the body has a difficult time healing any disease. Healing will not take place unless the two parts of the autonomic nervous system are in balance.

Color therapy can help achieve this balance. Researchers have documented that the red color spectrum can stimulate the sympathetic system. We do not need to use this color very often in therapy, since most of our life takes care of this very nicely. The color red is associated with anger, an increased heart rate, and an increase in blood pressure. The color blue, in contrast, will relax the sympathetic system and stimulate the parasympathetic system. This is the first step to healing disease. Think about how relaxing the blue ocean water and blue sky can be! A beach vacation can be very healing.

The College of Syntonics has investigated specific color wavelengths and studied their affects on eye disease. While this research is ongoing, the data to date indicate two promising findings: first, certain frequencies of blue-green light can improve vision in patients with macular degeneration; second, certain frequencies of green light can lower eye pressures in patients with glaucoma. The key here is "certain frequencies." Each color can have a myriad of frequencies and the color therapist's task is to identify the frequency of each color that best resonates with the patient's eye. This therapy can be compared to microcurrent stimulation, in microcurrent stimulation, specific frequencies of low currents are administered to the body to treat disease. Similar to microcurrent therapy, which relies on proper frequency selection, the success of color therapy treatment is based on selecting the proper color frequency for the patient.

Other physicians are joining the conversation, too. Dr. John Ott has found that the type of lighting that more closely simulates natural sunlight has a positive effect on health, behavior, and performance, while typical, artificial fluorescent light sources cause visual discomfort and lowered performance.

In 1985, psychiatrists discovered the benefits of light therapy. Now, in medical clinics throughout this country (and around the world), many individuals are receiving treatment for Seasonal Affective Disorder (SAD) in the form of exposure to bright light. People who are deprived of light for extended periods of time, such as those living in in northern latitudes during the winter, can develop this condition. SAD is characterized by depression, apathy, and low energy. We have already learned that the pineal gland is not being stimulated in this condition of light-deprivation; when it is not sufficiently stimulated, the pineal gland will not produce serotonin (the mood-elevating hormone) during the daylight hours. This deficiency leads to depression.

Light therapy is also commanding respect in the medical community for other reasons; currently, researchers are investigating its benefits as applied to treatment for jet lag, PMS, sleep disorders, and other conditions related to the body's daily rhythms. Researchers have found that exposure to certain colors can affect people's behaviors, moods, and physiological functions. Dr. Harry Wohlfarth, an authority on the effects of color on classroom performance, has found that lighting and colors chosen for walls and carpets in classrooms have a major influence on students' attendance, performance, and academic achievements. While we don't ordinarily think of classrooms as being healing environments, perhaps it is time we do so.

In 1991, Dr. Jacob Liberman's book, *Light: Medicine of the Future*, further expanded our understanding of light and color. The book describes the roles light and color play in creating a new experience of physical and emotional health. The following sections describe the colors used in light therapy and their effects.

RED

Red brings warmth, energy, and stimulation; therefore, it is good for low energy, fatigue, colds, chills, and passivity. Red activates people's energy. It raises intensity, exhilaration, activity levels, and passion. Slow and sluggish children should look at the color red before doing their homework. If it is used for an extended period of time over a few weeks or months, red color therapy will intensify your will and incentive to become physically active.

ORANGE

Orange is warm, cheering, and non-constricting. Orange acts upon the body and mind with freeing energy, relieving repressions. Subjects react to it strongly and intuitively. Orange creates cheerfulness and optimism; it clears people of weariness and listlessness, thereby increasing their ambition. Orange can improve the rhythm between waking and sleeping.

YELLOW

Yellow helps strengthen the nerves and the mind. It helps awaken mental inspiration and stimulates higher levels of mentality. Thus, it is an excellent color choice for people who are nervous or have nerve-related conditions or ailments. It makes people feel brightness and openness, due to its effect on the limbic brain. After looking at yellow, people find the urge to become intellectually active becomes stronger. Dissatisfied individuals soon change their facial expressions when they are exposed to yellow therapy.

GREEN

Green is the color of nature and the earth. In essence, it is balance and harmony, and possesses a soothing influence over both mind and body. Green enhances people's capacity for concentration. Unlike the deep, soothing sleepiness people experience when looking at blue light, green light gives people a type of relaxation that allows them to achieve a state of relaxed concentration. Green is the most neutralizing color. It detoxifies and cleanses.

BLUE

Blue is one of the greatest antiseptics in the world. It cools down inflammations and fever, lowers high blood pressure, stops bleeding, relieves bursting headaches, and calms strong emotions (like anger, aggression, or hysteria). It brings tranquility, soothes suffering, and conveys feelings of calm, silence, and restraint. Extended exposure to blue will create peaceful relaxation in people's bodies and make them feel a readiness to sleep. Blue helps ease tension headaches and restlessness. It also helps pressure in the stomach and cramps in the neck and spine disappear.

TURQUOISE

Turquoise has healing properties; it increases intuition and sensitivity. It works to disinfect people and can also be an antiseptic. Turquoise tones the general system, builds up the skin, and relaxes stressful sensations.

VIOLET

Violet is the color of transformation. It heals melancholy, hysteria, delusions, and alcohol addiction; it also brings spiritual insights and renewal. Shades of violet slow down an overactive heart and stimulate the spleen and the white blood cells (increasing immunity). Violet brings people to sleep; it soothes mental and emotional stress, and decreases sexual activity and sensitivity to pain. It helps in detoxification.

Leonardo da Vinci proclaimed that you can increase the power of meditation tenfold by meditating under the gentle rays of violet colors, as found in church windows. Violet helps to tune a person in to meditation and conveys inner strength, intuition, and inspiration to people.

Syntonic Light Therapy

Ocular—and general—phototherapy, often presented as Syntonic Light Therapy, has become one of the fastest-growing areas in clinical research and healthcare. How is a person evaluated for Syntonic Light Therapy, and how are colors selected for treatment?

I first became interested in Syntonic Light Therapy after I was invited to speak on homeopathy at an annual College of Syntonics meeting held in Santa Fe, New Mexico, in 2005. At that time, I was very skeptical of using light therapy. However, I wanted to learn more. While at the meeting, I asked a colleague to evaluate and treat me using light therapy. First, I underwent some baseline testing, which consisted of pupil, visual tracking, and color visual field evaluations. When I received the results, I was surprised to learn that I had difficulty tracking and that my visual fields were very constricted. I explained that these results could be due, in part, to my recent flight or to being at a high altitude—not to mention the stress of giving a major presentation at an international meeting. The therapist selected a color that matched my state and gave me a ten-minute treatment; then, I underwent the tests again. I could not believe the difference. My visual tracking had greatly improved, while my color visual fields had expanded by over 300 percent! After that, I became convinced that this color therapy was something I had to study and evaluate in order to use it to help my patients with their eye disease.

Thus, I began an earnest study of Syntonic Light Therapy under the guidance of my friends, Dr. Larry Wallace and Dr. Charles Butts. Dr. Wallace has used light therapy for over thirty-five years in treating chronic eye problems (including glaucoma, cataracts, and macular degeneration). In 2008, I became the first ophthalmologist to become a Fellow of the College of Syntonics.

I can still remember one of the very first patients I treated with Syntonic Light Therapy. A woman with advanced glaucoma, she was taking three different prescription eye drops, and her pressures were under very poor control. I evaluated her and treated her with light therapy for ten minutes. In thirty minutes, her pressures had been reduced from twenty-five to seventeen in both eyes!

Remember, the use of light therapy to treat glaucoma is not new. In 1948, the *American Journal of Ophthalmology* published an article that demonstrated certain spectrums of green light have a pressure-lowering affect on eyes with glaucoma. Much more recently, in May 2011, I published a paper, called "Homeopathic Syntonic Light Therapy in the Treatment of Glaucoma," in the *Journal of Optometric Phototherapy*. This paper reviewed the cases of eighteen patients who were treated with light therapy, and showed that all patients had a lowering of intraocular pressure after undergoing light therapy.

Cases of light therapy helping with macular degeneration have been as dramatic as in the glaucoma case described above. The most immediate effect of light therapy on patients with macular degeneration has been expansion of their visual fields. When people have macular degeneration, they experience a marked loss of central vision. If they have an associated loss of peripheral vision, then the patients do not have much useful vision left. Central vision plus peripheral vision equals functioning vision. I have seen patients experience a tremendous expansion of their visual fields almost immediately after undergoing color therapy. This translates, for them, into functioning vision that is much improved. However, I have not seen as marked an improvement of visual *acuity* using color therapy in patients with macular degeneration. It takes much longer to produce that type of result; often, additional treatments, such as microcurrent therapy and homeopathy, are needed.

In the March 1998 issue of the *Journal of Optometric Phototherapy*, an article called "Reversing Macular Degeneration," written by Sarah Cobb, makes some powerful points. She states that Syntonic Light Therapy not only improves vision but also improves patients' memories, as well as their overall vitality and reading skills.

Patients with cataracts can also benefit from Syntonic Light Therapy. I have also observed an immediate expansion of visual fields in patients with cataracts when using this therapy. As with treating macular degeneration, patients' improvement of acuity is often slower and they may still need additional therapies.

COLOR THERAPY AND BALANCING
THE NERVOUS SYSTEM

Syntonics comes from the word "syntony," or balance. We are concerned about the balance between the sympathetic and parasympathetic parts of the nervous system. When we have balance, we have health. If we have too much of the sympathetic, we go into fight or flight mode. If we have too much parasympathetic, then we can experience fatigue, digestive problems, sweating, and other difficulties. If you receive an eye evaluation as part of Syntonic Light Therapy, your evaluator will give special attention to the pupils, the action of the eye muscles, and the visual fields. This is because the pupils reflect the autonomic nervous system's balance in a very accurate manner.

Evaluating the pupils reveals, with great accuracy, whether there is balance in the autonomic system. When light shines into the eye, the pupil constricts, because of two factors: first, the stimulation of the parasympathetic nervous system; second, the corresponding relaxation of the sympathetic nervous system. When someone's pupils relax or dilate, this is because of stimulation of the sympathetic system and relaxation of the parasympathetic system. As you can see, there is interplay between the parasympathetic and sympathetic systems. In people who are in a balanced state, when light shines in their eyes, the pupils should constrict and *stay constricted*. If the pupils constrict but do not stay constricted (that is, if they then dilate), the patient has what are called alpha omega pupils. This indicates an imbalance, which can be of varying degrees, in the autonomic nervous system. Physicians evaluate the degree of alpha omega pupils on a scale of zero to four.

During a Syntonic Light Therapy evaluation, the practitioner will also examine the strength of the patient's eye muscles, looking especially at the eyes' ability to turn inward and outward. If someone is in a sympathetic state, the eyes tend to turn outward or look more to the periphery. To understand this, let's return to the example of fight or flight. If you are running away from a grizzly bear, you need good peripheral vision. In contrast, if someone is in a parasympathetic state the eyes tend to turn inward. For example, your eyes turn inward when you read; so, in order to read properly, you must be relaxed. So, light therapy practitioners evaluate the strength of the eyes' ability to turn inward and outward to evaluate the autonomic nervous system's balance once again.

The third set of measurements a practitioner takes during the evaluation is of the visual fields. The current method that most conventional eye doctors use to measure fields—and one that I believe is inadequate—is called "static perimetry." In this method, the patient puts his or her head in a fishbowl-like device, while lights flash in the periphery. If the patient can see the lights, he or she pushes a handheld button. However, I contend that this method is not physiological; our visual systems should be measured by using motion or movement, not by using flashing lights. In Syntonics, in contrast, we measure visual fields by using a kinetic (or motion-based) visual field test called a Campimeter. In this test, we move three distinctly colored objects in from the periphery of the patient's field of vision, and ask the patient to identify each color when it comes into his vision. This method both evaluates the visual field and also provides the practitioner with an energetic evaluation of the patient.

The Campimeter test uses, or "plots," three colors: red, green, and blue. During the test, the practitioner analyzes the color fields' size and shape in order to determine the person's physiological and emotional states. First, abnormalities found in reference to red, especially constriction of this color in the visual field, may indicate the presence of chronic health problems or chronic fatigue. This color may also reflect abnormalities in the circulatory system, high blood pressure, or diabetes. Second, since blue reflects more of the patient's psychological nature, abnormalities in perceiving blue might point to a patient having tension, migraine, headaches, sinus problems, or imbalances in the heart and adrenal systems. Third, constriction of green often indicates the patient has a focal infection or a systemic toxicity. These focal infections can affect the teeth, the tonsils, the sinuses, and the blood vessels of the eyes.

In order to understand the Syntonic approach to treating disease, let's look at the Syntonic Color Balance Beam. This balance beam represents the autonomic nervous system. On the left is the sympathetic system, or the red spectrum. On the right is the parasympathetic system, or the blue spectrum. In the center is green, which is the balance point. As I mentioned above, the goal of Syntonic Light Therapy is to help bring the autonomic nervous system into balance. After a therapist evaluates the patient and looks at the patient's pupil reaction, eye muscle balance, and colored visual fields, he or she determines the location of the patient's autonomic system on the balance beam and then selects a color to balance this system.

The basic Syntonic colors:

Alpha Delta (Red-Orange)

Patients who need this color for balance have Lazy Eye Syndrome; they have weak vision and poor focusing, and their eyes tend to turn inward.

Mu Delta (Yellow-Green)

Patients who require this color have Chronic Syndrome. Most people with long-standing eye problems will be in this category. A need for this color indicates chronic toxic, allergic, or neuroendocrine imbalances; it is very good in helping to detoxify the body.

Mu Upsilon (Blue-Green)

Patients who need this color have Acute Syndrome: they may have experienced recent head trauma, inflammations, or a high fever.

Upsilon Omega (Indigo)

Patients who require this color have Pain Reliever syndrome; they are experiencing headaches and eye discomfort.

Alpha Omega (Ruby)

Finally, Patients who need this color have Emotional Fatigue Syndrome. They may present with alpha omega pupils or be experiencing poor coping, mood swings, frustration, or adrenal fatigue.

I strongly believe light and color therapies are the prescriptions of the future. They are effective; they have no side effects or toxicity; and they are not only painless, but also pleasant to use. To learn more about the research in this field, which is going on all over the world, visit the International Light Association's website: www.international-light-association.org. or the College of Syntonic Phototherapy website: http://www.collegeofsyntonicoptometry.com/

Up to this point, we have covered all the basics or fundamentals required in order to establish the foundation for regaining health. These basics include proper diet, proper hydration, autonomic nervous system balance, and the establishment of optimal circadian rhythm (which provides better sleep at night and both energy and good moods during the day). These practices must be entered into as a whole; you must work on all of them at once. For example, if your autonomic nervous system is not balanced, you will not find sleeping in a dark room restful, because you will still be focused on your anxieties and worries. The good news is that the pineal gland is active in the daytime, continually producing serotonin, a substance that elevates moods and keeps depression at bay. So, fill your day with light in order to feel good; then, darken your surroundings at night in order to sleep well and protect your health.

CHAPTER SEVEN NOTES

Books

Liberman, Jacob. *Light: Medicine of the Future.* OD, Bear, and Company, 1999. Rochester, Vermont.

Ott, John. *Light, Radiation, and You: How to Stay Healthy.* Ariel Press, 1985. Atlanta, Georgia.

Notes

Eells, J.T., et al. "Photobiomodulation for the Treatment of Retinal Injury and Retinal Degenerative Diseases." In *Proceedings of Light-Activated Tissue Regeneration and Therapy Conference,* edited by R. W. Waynant and D. B. Tata, 39-51. New York: Springer, 2008.

Summary: Daily application of phototherapy (760 nanometers) in rodent subjects has been shown to prevent retinal injury following high-intensity laser burns and retinal toxicity due to methyl alcohol, as well as in cases of retinitis pigmentosa. Low energy levels of red and/or infrared light activates cytochrome oxidase, a photosensitive molecule in the mitochondria, which leads to an increase in retinal cellular activity, an increase in antioxidant properties, and an increase in general health and vitality.

The authors believe that the results of this study should prompt the FDA to approve these modalities for the treatment of macular degeneration and other eye diseases.

Ham, W.T., Jr., et al. "Action Spectrum for Retinal Injury from Near-Ultraviolet Radiation in the Aphakic Monkey." *American Journal of Ophthalmology* 93, no. (Mar. 1982): 299-306.

Pasternack, Bernard S. "Malignant Melanoma and Exposure to Fluorescent Lighting at Work." *The Lancet* 320, no. 8293 (7 August 1982): 290-3.

Rea, Mark. "Circadian Research." Presented at the International Conference on Light and Vision, Niagara Falls, Ontario, Canada. May 5-8, 2004.

Zaretskaya, R. B. "Intraocular Pressure of Normal and Glaucomatous Eyes as Affected by Accessory Light Stimuli." *American Journal of Ophthalmology* 31 (1948): 721-727.
Author's note: This is the first article I studied on the subject of glaucoma and light therapy.

Zhu, Yuan, Valter, Kristina, and J. Stone. "Environmental Damage to the Retina and Preconditioning: Contrasting Effects of Light and Hyperoxic Stress." *Investigative Ophthalmology & Visual Science* 51 (2010): 4821-4830.
Abstract: In this experiment one group of mice were raised in a normal light environment: twelve hours of light (3 lux) and twelve hours of darkness. Mice in the experimental group were exposed to bright light (300 lux) about 100 times brighter than normal room lighting. The mice were all exposed to retinal damaging light (1000 lux for two weeks) or plunged

into air-raised levels of oxygen. (High levels of oxygen are toxic to the retina.)

Author's note: Mice that were preconditioned to bright light did not have any retinal damage!

There are three possible mechanisms that allow preconditioning with light to protect the eye. Preconditioning stimulates healthy growth of key elements in the retina and increases antioxidant functioning. This preconditioning might have a beneficial effect in the treatment and prevention of progressive damage in macular degeneration and other eye diseases.

Websites

College of Syntonic Light Therapy

www.collegeofsyntonicoptometry.com

International Light Association

http://www.international-light-association.org

Microcurrent Stimulation

Microcurrent treatment is a technique that uses a very low current of electricity at a certain frequency to stimulate tissue and help heal or improve various vision problems: it is an important part of our practice. Studies show that this low-level current treatment, often referred to as simply "microcurrent," has many benefits for various physiological functions of the human body. Nearly one hundred published scientific articles discuss how microcurrent treatment improves circulation. Practitioners have healed cases of non-healing leg ulcers in diabetic patients using microcurrent and helped patients who have Raynaud's disease (a condition in which the fingers and the toes become blue and painful due to restricted peripheral vascular circulation). Microcurrent is used after tissue transplants and in plastic surgical procedures to improve circulation. There is no question that microcurrent can improve blood flow, and when blood flow is improved, nutrients can reach diseased areas to promote healing.

When my son, Sean, was young, he fell from a tree and broke a small bone on his wrist, the pisiform bone. This bone does not receive any blood flow, so the doctors working with Sean were concerned that it would not heal properly and cause a deformity that would affect his growth rate. The lack of blood flow was a major problem in healing. The doctors put him in a temporary cast just to see what would happen; however, they were not very optimistic and predicted he would need surgery when the cast came off. In the interim, I applied microcurrent constantly to Sean's break. When the doctors removed the cast and took an X-ray, they were surprised to see that the bone was completely healed. Orthopedic surgeons now routinely use microcurrent for healing certain fractures and joints.

Microcurrent treatment also stimulates cellular activities. For example, Dr. Ngok Cheng, a Korean researcher, published a paper on his studies of the effects of different current levels on rats' skin cells in the *Journal of Clinical Orthopedic Research*. He applied various levels of current and performed blood analysis to measure the effects of the different currents on blood chemistry. His study showed dramatic improvement in protein synthesis and, even more significantly, showed that the cells' ATP (adenosine triphosphate) activity increased up to 500 percent. ATP is very important because it is like gasoline for cells; the more you have of it, the better your cells work. We are not talking

5 percent, 10 percent, or 20 percent, which would all be statistically significant; we are talking about 500 percent, which is an amazing increase in cellular activity.

LESS IS MORE

In the study described above, Dr. Cheng also found that when he applied a higher level of current, the cellular activity actually decreased. This is where the real caution comes in: therapy is an art. We are talking about using *micro*currents, not larger currents. Once you start using above 500 microamps, and go up to 1,000 microamps—in particular, when you get to about 1,000 microamps—cellular activity decreases. One more thing you have to understand is that therapists must consider more than just the amount of current being delivered to the tissue; they must also consider the surface area's size. Delivering 1,000 amps to a large area is different than delivering 1,000 amps to a pinpoint. Therefore, surface area and current strength need to be calibrated precisely.

Many of the microcurrent machines on the market have a small knob on them that allows the patient to adjust the current during treatment. I think those types of machines can be dangerous, especially when they are used for treating the eye. Turning the current up too high could affect optical nerve activity; it could possibly cause a decrease in vision and harm the eye. This is one of the reasons the FDA has stated microcurrent should not be used on the eye. Many of the early microcurrent machines delivered only high current levels.

However, now we have new equipment that is calibrated to deliver the right amount of current to delicate eye tissues. To understand this idea, let's use the metaphor of gardening. I am a gardener, so I know that when I have tiny seedlings I have to be very careful watering them. I don't want to subject them to a blast of water; I want them to have a light mist. These seedlings are like the retina's delicate structures. Just as a blast of water from the garden hose will destroy the seedlings, a high electrical current applied to the retina will harm those delicate tissues.

Even misting seedlings with water has to be regulated, and this regulation occurs through resistance. If my neighbor comes over and steps on the garden hose I'm using, what is going to happen? That mist is going to decrease. That's because the pressure of his foot on the garden hose has increased the resistance. A similar effect happens when current is applied to skin; the body has resistance that determines how much current will flow into it. The more resistance there is on your skin, the less flow occurs. What determines resistance on your skin? There are many factors, including your hydration level, your mineral content, and so forth. Everybody has a different level of resistance and, in fact, that resistance is changing constantly. As the resistance decreases, you will have more flow. This continual change in resistance is why adjustments must be made. In this, the machine is like the garden hose; if my neighbor steps on the garden hose and the flow of water decreases, I can go to the faucet and turn it up. In the microcurrent machine, the voltage or the battery is equivalent to a faucet. The voltage, the resistance, and the current in the flow constantly interact.

When a therapist uses the microcurrent machine, he or she makes constant adjustments to the battery or the voltage to determine a steady current or flow. This continuous flow is essential for both beneficial results and safety. Remember, when the current is too high, the therapy can actually reduce the cellular activity.

Ideally, a therapist wants to use around 40 microamps on retinal tissue. When I first started to do microcurrent therapy, I used about 400 microamps. According to my allopathic mind, more was better. Over the years, however, I have decreased the levels I use in therapy, and I am getting better results. First, I went from 400 to 100; now, I do 40 and, on some people, I reduce to 20. I am using less and less microcurrent.

Once, I was discussing microcurrent treatment with several very skeptical doctors and I explained how I had been using less current and getting better results. One doctor said, "Dr. Kondrot, if less gives you better results, just don't do it at all, and you will get the best outcome!" His statement showed that he failed to understand the basic laws of healing illustrated by homeopathic principles. Homeopaths want to stimulate the body to heal gently. Just because food is good, we don't want to eat one hundred meals a day! Seedlings need water, but too much water will kill them. All things in excess can be harmful.

I know of a brilliant microcurrent therapist from Hong Kong, Millie Ning, who is doing amazing work on people who have structural problems. She treats conditions like scoliosis, deformity of the big toe, and so on, using only ten microamps of current. As a result, I am considering reducing the amount of current even more in my own work. What I am observing in microcurrent is a homeopathic law. In homeopathy, the greater the dilution, the better the effect. I think that microcurrent, like homeopathy, uses subtle energy: less is not less, but is actually more.

HOW GOLF LEAD ME TO MICROCURRENT THERAPY

I began using microcurrent about fifteen years ago after reading an article about Sam Snead, the famous golfer. Snead had experienced really beneficial effects from undertaking microcurrent therapy for his macular degeneration. After reading the article about him, I phoned the microcurrent machine manufacturer and ordered ten machines. I then contacted ten of my patients who had macular degeneration—patients who were not doing well—and I treated every one of them with microcurrent. I was pleasantly surprised when eight out of the ten did better, and started regularly using microcurrent in my practice as a result.

I think this is the way that medicine should be practiced: A doctor makes an observation about a method or treatment, and then he or she duplicates it. If the duplication works, then he or she incorporates the method into his or her practice. Unfortunately, now it's the pharmaceutical companies that practice medicine. The average doctor waits for a national, controlled study that shows that a method or drug works before trying it. I do not believe medicine is supposed to be practiced this way. Medicine should empower thousands of doctors to observe methods and treatment, and trust their observations, so they can develop their art and help their patients.

Now, I want to return to my story about Sam Snead. After using microcurrent in my practice for some time, I had the opportunity to treat Sam Snead. I flew down to his home in Florida, stayed with him for a week, and treated him. I think at that time he was in his early eighties, and he was amazingly flexible. He consented to give me golf lessons. The first couple of days, he took me out to the range with a bucket of balls and looked at my swing. He finally came up to me, put his arm around me, and said, "Dr. Kondrot, here is my advice. I want you to cut back on golf for a year, and then I want you to just give it up."

My treatment helped Sam improve his vision. At that time, he was under the supervision of his family doctor, who said to me, "If I were not here to observe this [his improvement], I would have doubted that he would have any improvement in his vision."

Sam was quoted as saying, "I am going to get a driver's license next year."

Sam is not the only athlete to benefit from microcurrent therapy. In addition to improving blood flow and increasing cellular activity, microcurrent can remove scar tissue. Many professional athletes are now receiving microcurrent to help in their rehabilitation. For example, Dr. Carolyn McMakin popularized microcurrent among athletes by working with famous football players Bill Romanowski and Terrell Owens. In fact, when Terrell Owens injured his ankle in 2005, doctors predicted he would take eighteen months to heal. After receiving FSM (Frequency Specific Microcurrent) treatment, he played in the Super Bowl six weeks later. Physicians of teams in the NHL, the NBA, and the NFL—as well as the U.S. Postal Service Pro Cycling Team (Lance Armstrong's former team)—have all used FSM therapy. Many chronic injuries clear up in record time. Nerve injuries, inflammation, and scar tissue all appear to respond well to the treatment; what's more, microcurrent has no side effects. I talked with Lance Armstrong's doctor, who told me he travels with numerous microcurrent machines. In one race, Lance suffered a hairline fracture in his ankle. He should have been out for the entire racing season, but they rehabilitated his ankle at night using microcurrent.

EQUIPMENT IMPROVED

Microcurrent treatment and microcurrent equipment have changed significantly since 1998. Many eye patients become interested in microcurrent after reading my book, *Microcurrent Stimulation: Miracle Eye Cure*, and they expect to experience the same type of equipment and treatment outlined in the book when they go in for microcurrent treatment. However, the equipment and treatment have both evolved since that book was published. I hope this report will give you a much better understanding of how they have changed in the interim.

I began using one type of equipment, the Microstim 100, in 1998. This single-channel machine had four fixed frequencies and used a probe to treat eight acupuncture points around the eye (four points above and four below each eye). The machine treated each point for twelve seconds, using four different frequency settings (292 Hz, 30 Hz, 9.1 Hz and 0.3 Hz). These specific frequencies came from the research of the late French neurologist Dr. Paul Nogier, who is best known for his innovative work in the development of auriculotherapy (ear acupuncture). Through his research, Dr. Nogier developed frequencies for increasing blood flow, reducing inflammation, and assisting in general healing. Research suggested that the higher frequencies, 292 and 30 Hz, reduced inflammation while the lower frequencies, 9.1 Hz and 0.3 Hz, helped stimulate healing.

I published data concerning the use of this instrument in treatment in 2001, in my book *Microcurrent Stimulation: Miracle Eye Cure*, and in October 2002 in the *Townsend Letter* (a peer-reviewed journal about natural therapies).

However, the Microstim 100 and its probe had several disadvantages. First, treating eight points around the eye with a probe was a cumbersome task. Many macular degeneration patients had difficulty locating these points on their own; treatment also became difficult, because keeping the probe fixed on these points required a steady hand and good vision. The machine also had a current adjustment knob. The machine's instructions told patients to turn up the current until they felt a tingling, and then reduce the current until they felt nothing. Many patients treated their eyes with current levels that were much too high; because of this, the results were very unpredictable. Later, the manufacturers modified the Microstim 100 into a delivery system that came with eyeglasses. However, this system still had two limitations: patients could adjust the current and the current delivery was unpredictable. The key to success in microcurrent treatment is to keep the current at a low level. However, it is human nature to turn the current up higher, because we usually think that more is better.

After using the Microstim 100 for a while, I had a discussion with Dr. Jim Suzuki, an electrical engineer and president of the Biotherapeutics Company, that led me to investigate a two-channel microcurrent machine his company had developed. This machine had two separate channels and a frequency offset of 0.7 Hz. This means the company developed the machine using the basic Nogier frequencies but used an offset of 0.7 Hz: (292/292.7 Hz, 30/30.7 Hz, 9.1/9.8 Hz, and 0.3/1.0 Hz). The company theorized that this delivery system would produce a range of frequencies that could be absorbed by the body more readily. Similar to a broad-spectrum antibiotic, this machine offered a broad-spectrum effect and could have a much greater therapeutic effect as a result. This machine had the advantage of using a fixed current (at 100 microamps), regardless of the resistance present in the patient's body.

Dr. Suzuki helped me develop a delivery system for the machine that had patients use eyeglasses, but the glasses were eventually discontinued because of manufacturing problems, as well as problems with delivering consistent currents into the eye. Still, this machine had two distinct advantages in the fixed current's increased safety and the dual-channel delivery system's broader action. When using this machine, patients could not increase the current to dangerous levels.

Improved Equipment and Techniques

The Frequency Specific Microcurrent (FSM) technique, which I discussed earlier in relation to athletes using microcurrent, has produced dramatic improvement in macular degeneration treatment outcomes. Instead of using basic, generic frequencies (which have a low-level effect on the diseased tissue), now, with FSM, we can use two different frequency channels to deliver both tissue frequency and pathology frequency.

Let me explain this concept. Each tissue has a specific frequency, or vibration, as does each type of pathology. This frequency depends on the area's hydration, density, molecular structure, amounts of carbon and hydrogen, nitrogen bonding, and so forth. For example, bone tissue would have a different frequency than skin or heart tissue, while scar tissue would have a different frequency than tissue that was swollen. For comparison's sake, look at a musical tuning fork. If you have a tuning fork with a frequency of the note "C," it will vibrate according to that frequency. If you have two tuning forks with "C" frequencies and vibrate them together, they will support each other and vibrate in harmony. However, if you then take the same "C"-frequency tuning fork and vibrate it next to a "D"-frequency tuning fork, you will have disharmony; in fact, the frequencies might cancel each other out.

Another example is that of an opera singer who hits the right frequency of a nearby crystal glass, at a very high volume, and the glass shatters. This is because the frequency of the singer's voice matched the frequency of the glass, which produced the shattering effect. Of course, we don't want to shatter tissues with frequencies. That's why we use very low currents to delivery frequencies to the tissue. When we match the treatment frequencies to the tissue frequencies, we achieve a supportive harmony that acts as a mechanism to help strengthen and heal the tissue.

Now, let's look at the type of channel used to treat pathology. We obviously don't want a frequency to harmonize and strengthen the pathology's frequency, so this machine delivers frequencies that are disharmonious to the pathology in order to weaken the pathology's effect.

The roots of FSM treatment date back to the early 1900s and to Dr. Albert Abrams, the first physician to use calibrated instruments capable of detecting living tissue's radiations. Dr. Abrams concluded that all matter radiates electromagnetic energy, and that the characteristics of each type of radiation depend upon the matter's unique molecular structure. Dr. Carolyn McMakin, a chiropractor, has expanded the range of Modern FSM by studying hundreds of different frequencies within the range of .01 to 999 Hz, with varying intensities of 20 to 600 microamps. Her work supports Dr. Abrams' findings, confirming that each of the body's tissues has an individualized frequency. For example, the retina's frequency is 95 Hz and the macula's is 137 Hz. Each type of pathology also has a frequency. A hemorrhage has a frequency of 18 Hz, while an edema's is 14 Hz. FSM treatment is "frequency specific" because the tissue's frequencies and the pathology's frequencies are "matched" against two frequencies in the FSM machine. For example, suppose a practitioner is treating a patient with a hemorrhage in the macula. The FSM treatment would use 18 Hz (for the hemorrhage) and 137 Hz (for the macula). This set of coupled frequencies matches the exact abnormalities present in the damaged tissue. The desired effect of the treatment is a neutralization of the frequencies that are in disharmony.

After learning about FSM research, I began using a special FSM machine, the Precision Microcurrent machine, to treat all my eye patients. This machine's technology delivers two distinct channels of current and specific frequencies during treatment, and these channels can be programmed to match a patient's tissue and pathology frequencies. With this machine, I began treating patients with thirty to forty separate frequency pairs. I applied each frequency pair for a duration of one minute, and achieved much better results than the results gained when using the single channel probe with four Nogier frequencies. Using this new method, I noticed that the results increased; instead of 60 percent, over 80 percent of patients experienced an improvement. The average patient's vision improvement increased from gaining one-half or one line on the eye chart to gaining over two lines.

The Need of a Machine for Home Use

I had one problem with this therapy, though. After treating patients with these frequency pairs and seeing such good results, I could not send them home with this device to continue self-treatment. The machines are expensive (costing over $8,000) and require someone to operate them, changing frequency pairs every minute. This type of operation is not an easy task, especially if you have poor vision. As an interim plan, my office sent patients home with the machines that have four Nogier frequencies. These machines are much more affordable and can still be used to help maintain results. We suggested that the patients then return every three to six months to repeat the specific frequency pairs with our FSM machine.

In the meantime, I became interested in developing a low-cost, portable, programmable microcurrent machine that patients could take home with them. I wanted to develop a machine that had specific frequency pair measurements and could be effective for their particular eye problems.

I started consulting several electrical engineering firms in the United States, but my initial meetings were not very promising. Typically, the firms wanted $20,000 to $30,000 just to do a feasibility study. Even then, the engineers I met were very skeptical about their ability to design such a machine and then have it pass FDA usage standards. I was very depressed and discouraged, but I still believed that a machine like this must be developed.

Back to School for Dr. K.!

I then decided to take the bull by the horns, so to speak, and called up the Department Chair of the Arizona State School of Electrical Engineering. I told him I wanted to go back to school and get a master's degree in Electrical Engineering. "What in the world are you doing here?" was his initial reaction. Despite this feedback, the department accepted me into the program. My first class was Advanced Digital Circuits, which I thought would be the class that held all the answers. It turns out I was in over my head, but

I still began to meet the right people—people who could possibly help me with my engineering project.

During this time, I met Ning Wu, a brilliant, third-generation electrical engineer whose father is an electrical engineering professor at Beijing University. Thanks to the brilliant work of Ning Wu and his team of electrical engineers, we were able to develop the first programmable microcurrent machine for home use.

This machine has five specific programs that can be customized for each patient; each program can be customized with frequency pairs specific to each patient's eye problem. Now, patients can take customized protocols home with them and get continued benefit from the treatments. (We design these programs not only to treat the eye, but also to detoxify the body, reduce stress, and treat other physical problems.)

The machine delivers current through silver mesh gloves, which are wrapped in a damp washcloth. We find that this method is much easier for patients to use than a probe. Patients can sit back, relax, and apply the delivery system by using a moist washcloth to cover their eyes. After testing, this delivery system has demonstrated the ability to deliver microcurrent energy into the eye consistently. Because the gloves and washcloths are versatile, the machine can also aid in detoxification and all-over body programs.

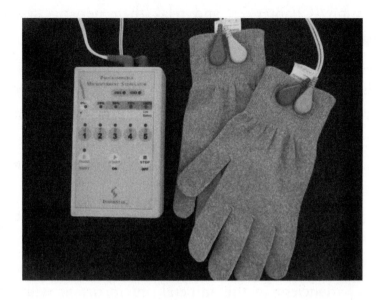

It is very important that patients interested in micro-current receive this treatment under the supervision of an eye doctor experienced in microcurrent use. This is one reason why, at our practice, we have established the three-day treatment program called "Healing the Eye." In this program, each day, patients receive two to four microcurrent treatments while we carefully monitor the state of their eyes. This method is especially helpful for glaucoma patients; microcurrent can be extremely benefi-cial for treating glaucoma because it helps lower pressure and improve circulation to the optic nerve. Most glaucoma patients who undergo microcurrent will see an improve-ment in their visual fields and vision after just three days of treatment.

Remember, microcurrent is not a miracle eye cure. In order to obtain the best results, I firmly believe patients need to make dietary changes (see Chapter 1), improve hydration (Chapter 2), and relax their nervous systems (Chapter 3). When all these factors are addressed, the patients' eyes will be more receptive to microcurrent's healing power. It is also important that, before undergoing microcurrent treatment, you ask the following questions:

1. Will an eye professional monitor me during the first few treatments? Is this person an ophthalmologist or optometrist?

2. Have my health and nutritional state been evaluated (before beginning)?

3. Have my zinc levels been evaluated? (If you are deficient in this mineral, microcurrent will have little effect!)

4. What is the current level and frequency of the microcurrent machine that will be used? (Some settings on microcurrent machines can actually make your vision worse.)

Microcurrent can play an important role in helping you improve your vision. By using it, I have helped thousands of patients who are suffering from macular degeneration, glaucoma, and cataracts. Consider healing your eye the natural way, through the use of this amazing technology, without resorting to surgery, injections, or harmful drugs.

MY PERSONAL STORY

On Sunday, October 3, 2011, I finished the Marine Corps Marathon in Washington, D.C., along with my wife and stepson (Ly and Lawrence). It had been twenty years since I had run a marathon, and, at the age of sixty, I should have trained properly before attempting the race. Unfortunately, due to my busy schedule, I only completed a few ten-mile runs as part of my training. In my prime, over twenty years previously, I typically ran sixty to eighty miles a week.

When I reached the twenty-mile mark, I felt like I was dying, and, after finishing the race, my body was incredibly sore. Forget walking! I was only able to shuffle, and I had to slide my body in and out of bed. Ly and Lawrence were just as sore. Ly and I took some homeopathic *Arnica*, which relieved the pain, but the soreness persisted.

The following night, we decided to do a microcurrent treatment for the muscle soreness. My favorite way of doing this is to sit in a hot tub and let the healing current flow through the water. You might be wondering: How does this work? Doesn't the current short out in the water—before reaching the body? Well, I use FSM, and the current carries specific frequencies that match body tissues and pathologic conditions. The way this works is during the microcurrent treatment, specific frequencies or vibrations, formed by the microcurrent machine, resonate into the water and are then transfered into the person sitting in the water. This resonation harmonizes with the particular tissues and problems that need to be treated. In this case, I used frequencies specific to inflammation, pain, and toxins. When the correct frequency vibrates with a tissue, it will harmonize the tissue and stimulate healing.

To my surprise after a thirty-minute treatment, both Ly and I were back to normal. I was absolutely stunned! Even twenty years ago, with proper training, I would be sore for at least a week after running a marathon. This miracle has reinforced my belief in microcurrent's power to treat inflammation, acute and chronic disease, and eye disease.

SUMMARY OF MICROCURRENT'S EFFECTS

Because this chapter contains more technical information than the previous chapters, the essential information about microcurrent therapy is summarized below.

Microcurrent Works in Five Ways

- Improves circulation
- Stimulates cellular activity
- Reduces inflammation
- Removes scar tissue
- Achieves a neuroprotective effect

Some of Microcurrent's Miraculous Effects

- Proven track record of healing tissues, muscles, bones, and specific organs
- Unparalleled ability to treat pain
- Rejuvenation of the skin, the organs, and the body
- Resonance effect: Frequencies can be matched to the body, helping to heal physical and emotional disharmony.

CHAPTER EIGHT NOTES

Newsletters and Magazines

"Can Macular Degeneration be Reversed?" *The Lion,* (Dec. 2001-Jan. 2002).

"Clinical Discoveries: New Treatment for Macular Degeneration." Robert Rowen, *Second Opinion Newsletter* (August 2002): 6-8.

Research Articles and Publications

Microcurrent Improves Vascular Circulation

Debreceni, L., Gyulai, M., Debreceni, A., and K. Szabo. "Results of Transcutaneous Electrical Stimulation (TES) In Cure of Lower Extremity Arterial Disease." *Angiology* 46 (1995): 613-618.

Kaada, B. "Vasodilation Induced By Transcutaneous Nerve Stimulation In Peripheral Ischemia (Raynaud's Phenomenon and Diabetic Polyneuropathy)." *European Heart Journal* 3 (1982): 303-314.

---. "Promoted Healing of Chronic Ulceration by Transcutaneous Nerve Stimulation (TNS)." *Vasa* 12 (1983): 262-269.

Kjartansson, J., and T. Lundberg. "Effects of Electrical Nerve Stimulation (ENS) In Ischemic Tissue." *Scandinavian Journal of Plastic and Reconstructive Surgery and Hand Surgery* 24 (1990): 129-134.

Microcurrent Improves Cellular Activity

Cheng, Ngok. "The Effects of Electrical Current on ATP Generation, Protein Synthesis, and Membrane Transport In Rat Skin." *Clinical Orthopedics and Related Research* 171 (Nov. - Dec. 1982): 264-271.

Microcurrent and Macular Degeneration

Kondrot, Edward C. *Microcurrent Stimulation: Miracle Eye Cure.* Berkeley, CA: North Atlantic Books, 1999.

Initial Results of Microcurrent Stimulation in the Treatment of Age-Related Macular Degeneration, Edward Kondrot, Townsend Letter- Pages 65- 67, October 2002.

Michael, Leland D., and Merrill J. Allen. "Nutritional Supplementation, Electrical Stimulation, and Age-Related Macular Degeneration." *Journal of Orthomolecular Medicine* 8, no. 3 (Third Quarter, 1993).

Miller, Damon P. *The Treatment of Macular Degeneration, Stargardt's Disease, Retinitis Pigmentosa, and Other Retinal Disease with Microcurrent Stimulation Therapy.* 2000. Posted on web site http://www.acupunctureworks.organicmd.com/macular/first120.htm

Microcurrent and Retinitis Pigmentosa

Pagani, Lucia, Manni, Luigi, and Luigi Aloe. "Effects of Electroacupuncture on Retinal Nerve Growth Factor and Brain-Derived Neurotrophic Factor Expression In a Rat Model of Retinitis Pigmentosa." Available online 11 May 2006. Brain Research, 1092 (2006), 198-206. *Abstract: The study revealed that daily sessions of low-frequency electro- acupuncture during a critical developmental stage of retinal cell degeneration cause an increase of in in protective elements in the eye which might slow the progression of retinitis pigmentosa.*

Microcurrent and Glaucoma

MCS lowers eye pressure.

Chu, Teh-Ching and David E. Potter. "Ocular Hypotension Induced by Electroacupuncture," *Journal of Ocular Pharmacology and Therapeutics* 18, no. 4 (2002): 293- 305.

This study, published by Teh-Ching Chu in the Journal of Ocular Pharmacology, shows that electroacupuncture (EA) lowered intraocular pressures in rabbits. The purpose of the study was to examine the effects of electroacupuncture on intraocular pressure in rabbits. Researchers performed EA stimulation through acupuncture needles placed close to the sciatic nerve at points located at GB-30 or gallbladder 30, selecting these points because they offered greater precision in terms of needle placement. The study revealed that the placement of the needle in an acupuncture meridian is critical. Placement of needles in non-acupuncture point areas were not that effective in lowering eye pressure. During the study, researchers found the intraocular pressure was decreased as much as 9 mm Hg, and lasted for more than nine hours.

This study confirms my observation that microcurrent can lower intraocular pressure, which is observed in patients after they receive MCS treatment. I believe that an even more important effect of microcurrent is the increase in blood flow to the optic nerve it provides. Most eye doctors will agree that glaucoma's main destructive component is not an increase in eye pressure but a decrease in optic nerve circulation, which makes the nerve susceptible to variations in eye pressure.

www.healingtheeye.com/PDF/EA Glaucoma_pressure.pdf

Evidence: Microcurrent Has a Neuroprotective Effect in the Treatment of Glaucoma

Chan, H.H., et al. "Electroacupuncture Provides a New Approach to Neuroprotection in Rats with Induced Glaucoma." *The Journal of Alternative and Complementary Medicine* 11, no. 2 (April 2005): 315-322.

This article, published in *The Journal of Alternative and Complementary Medicine,* was based on research done at the Department of Optometry and Radiology at Hong Kong Polytechnic University.

Researchers used laser photocoagulation to induce glaucoma in the right eyes of fourteen adult rats. (This causes scarring and build-up of glaucoma pressure in the eye.) They used the rats' left eyes as a control. Then, researchers divided the animals into three groups. One group received no treatment; the second group received electroacupuncture treatment at 2 Hz; and the third group received electroacupuncture treatment at 100 Hz. Researchers performed three treatment sessions each week for four weeks and studied the rats' visual function using electroretinalgram measurements (ERG).

Researchers showed there was no neuroprotection in the untreated group or the group that received treatment at 100 Hz. In the group that received treatment at 2 Hz wave form, researchers observed a retinal protective effect when measuring changes in the retinal waveforms.

The study's authors concluded that electroacupuncture at a rate of 2 Hz provides neuroprotection in rats by preserving their retinal function. Based on such results, low-frequency EA treatment may be an alternative therapy for glaucoma treatment.

I have been using microcurrent to treat glaucoma since 1999. I believe its mechanism of action is threefold: it improves blood flow, stimulates cellular activity, and reduces inflammation and scar tissue. Now, we have research evidence that microcurrent has a protective effect on the optic nerve. Why is this important? The problem with glaucoma is not so much the pressure in the eye itself, but the effect that pressure has on blood flow to the optic nerve. Patients with glaucoma have a compromised optic nerve. Elevations in pressure can cause the optic nerve's blood flow to be reduced, resulting in damage to the nerve and loss of vision. This is why microcurrent can be so beneficial to patients with glaucoma. This therapy helps to increase blood flow and stimulate cellular activity, and now we have evidence that it also provides a neuroprotective effect.

www.healingtheeye.com/PDF/EA_Neuroprotective_ Glaucoma.pdf

Websites

www.microcurrentconference.org
www.inspirstar.com
www.frequencyspecific.com

CHAPTER 9

Specialized Therapies

This chapter provides you with a host of additional ways to boost healing and improve vision—that is, after you have changed your diet, become hydrated, and learned to relax. You do not need to think about doing all of them, but consider selecting one or two that seem to resonate with your needs.

NUTRITIONAL INTRAVENOUS THERAPIES

We discussed intravenous nutritional therapy, focusing especially on the Myers' Cocktail, in Chapter 1. This type of therapy bears mentioning again in this chapter, which is devoted to therapies that deliver targeted, intense, short-term boosts of energy to cells and tissues to stimulate their healing potential. Patients who have not had "proper nutrition" (and by that I mean organic, whole foods) for most of their lives *all* need to boost their nutritional status in order for any of the other therapies they undergo to be maximally effective.

Another form of intravenous supplementation uses vitamin C. This method involves the administration of high doses of the water-soluble vitamin, far beyond what the patient can take orally, and it has been used with some success in cataract treatment.

Myers' Cocktail

As discussed in Chapter 1, this is one of the most commonly used IV therapies. It has a high concentration of vitamin C, B-complex vitamins, taurine, trace minerals, and zinc. Receiving it is one of the best ways to jumpstart your body's nutritional state. In fact, we recommend patients receive this therapy during our three-day eye health program; we also suggest patients undergoing microcurrent treatment receive a Myers' Cocktail once a month. Myers' Cocktail is also very helpful for recovery after illness or injury.

Patricia Kane's Protocol

Patricia Kane, whom I introduced earlier, believes if a person supports the cell membrane with good nutrition, the cell will function optimally, resulting in excellent neurological function. This belief is supported by the results she has achieved in over thirty years of helping patients with neurological problems. She is truly a miracle worker who treats the most advanced neurological cases with amazing results. Five years before writing this book, I attended one of her seminars, so I could learn her amazing techniques and use them to help eye patients. Because the eye is part of the neurological system, anything that benefits the neurological system will help the eye and vision; so, Kane's techniques have benefited many patients with glaucoma, optic nerve problems, and macular degeneration. My friend, Dr. Dennis Courtney, encouraged me to retake her course this year, since many new developments had taken place in the field in the past five years. All the while, Kane has been advancing her research and perfecting her treatments to get better results.

Let's look at the cell membrane in the retina and see how correct nutrition, especially the inclusion of proper lipids, is essential to maintaining vision and restoring lost vision. The retina has 100 million rods and cones. Each rod or cone has a stack of lipid membrane with up to 2,000 layers. The surface area of all the membranes in the retina is about forty square miles. That is a great deal of lipid surface area. In each stack of the lipid membrane are 140 million rhodopsin molecules. Rhodopsin molecules are responsible for capturing photons and producing sight.

Each day, every retinal receptor cell discards about 6 to 7 percent of these membranes. In addition, each day it must reconstitute these membranes, along with 10 million new rhodopsin molecules. The entire photo-receiving system is renewed every fourteen days. In other words, you have a new retina every two weeks. Clearly, if you don't have the right nutrition, the retinal function will decline rapidly.

In fact, if you don't ingest the proper lipids for renewing these retinal membranes, you could experience a total loss of vision in just fourteen days.

What are these lipids that are so essential for retinal renewal? The retina's membranes are 50 to 55 percent docosahexaenoic acid (DHA), which is an omega-3 fatty acid. DHA's highest concentration in the body is inside the eye. In order for the eye's cells to utilize DHA in the best possible way, researchers have found that the body needs a four-to-one ratio of fatty acids (four units of omega 6 to one unit of omega 3). We discussed the importance of omega oils for overall health and nutrition in the first chapter; now, we see how important they are for eye health. Another very important lipid for cell function is phosphatidylcholine (PC), which makes up close to 60 percent of the cell membrane, and helps to keep the ratio of DHA at the optimal level of four to one.

Kane has developed a PC intravenous protocol for treating devastating neurological health disorders; this protocol uses IV lipid therapy and oral fatty acid supplementation. Her protocols have yielded marked positive responses in the treatment of severe neurological disorders such as ALS, Parkinson's, multiple sclerosis, Alzheimer's, autism, pervasive developmental delay, seizure disorders, post-stroke disorders, traumatic brain injuries, and metabolic and genetic abnormalities.

From Kane, I learned that intravenous PC passes through the blood-brain barrier. This is important to know since, for any treatment to be effective on the retina, it must pass this blood-brain barrier. Notably, many conventional drugs do not pass this barrier. Kane's PC IV protocol can also aid in the removal of heavy metals. In fact, Kane has been using PC IV protocols to treat cases of heavy metal poisoning. She believes that PC is more effective and less toxic than conventional EDTA chelation, since EDTA does not readily pass the blood-brain barrier.

When used intravenously, PC can also act as a carrier and help other agents to pass the blood-brain barrier. Kane's protocol includes the IV administration of glutathione, a very powerful antioxidant. When administered alongside the PC, more of the glutathione passes into the brain and the eye, and it has a much greater therapeutic effect than when it is administered alone.

One recent development in the field is an oral form of PC. Now, I am making the oral PC form part of the vitamin protocol our office prescribes to patients with macular degeneration, glaucoma, and cataracts. (If you are interested in PC supplementation, make sure to avoid using PC made from lecithin. To make lecithin, people degum crude soy oil, bleach it, and then later process it by adding oil. PC made from lecithin is ineffective and will be broken down into its component parts when it enters the body.)

I have been using Kane's PC protocol for the past five years to treat patients with degenerative disorders of the eye; in particular, I use it with patients who have macular degeneration and glaucoma. After hearing about Kane's latest research, I will be revising my protocol to implement it and help you save your vision.

OXIDATIVE THERAPIES

Oxidative therapies, which include an assortment of techniques and protocols, add more oxygen to your cells, thereby stimulating healing and optimal functioning. Accepted methods of oxidative therapies include ozone, hydrogen peroxide, and ultraviolet light therapies. They all produce charged oxygen molecules and have similar reactions in the body.

Ultraviolet Light Therapy

I introduced this technique in the earlier chapter on sleep and light. Ultraviolet light therapy is another of technique that energizes a patient's metabolic processes quickly while reducing or eliminating infections. (These infections drain an organism and compromise its potential to mount a good immune response to current problems.) Many eye conditions can be addressed like the other diseases that follow low vitality, poor lifestyle choices, bad diet, increased stress, and environmental toxins. At our practice's three-day eye program, we routinely use oxidative therapies. Each patient receives a minimum of two oxidative IV therapies during "Healing the Eye." Since beginning this therapy, I have observed an increase in the overall visual improvement of patients who attend the three-day program.

Oxygen Therapy

We may be able to last a month or more without food, while we can only make it a few days without water. However, we can only survive for a few minutes without oxygen. Oxygen, which is carried by the blood, suffuses all the cells in the body every second. Without it, there is nearly instant death. We all keep breathing, which seems to keep everything working pretty well. However, we may as well acknowledge that people who have chronic diseases have cells that are at least partially deprived of oxygen. If you have an acute disease or infection, there is probably a pretty serious oxygen deficit in your tissues, too. If so, you have entered a situation that is beyond repair by exercise or deep breathing. It requires oxygen therapy.

Oxygen therapy is the addition of oxygen molecules to your tissues in order to make them healthy and more functional. The body can receive the molecules through a variety of administration procedures. One amazing thing about this therapy is that it works almost instantaneously, while the effects can last for some time. The other amazing thing about this therapy is that even though people started practicing it decades ago, with great results, it still has not found its rightful place in conventional medicine. A researcher named Emmett Knott first discovered the effectiveness of oxygen therapy on seriously and moderately ill patients. He treated the blood of his first human subject in 1928. The patient had a case of sepsis (bloodstream infection) following an abortion. She had been declared beyond help by the attending physicians, but responded dramatically to the therapy. He treated many other patients with bacterial infections and viruses, and some were comatose—many of them were close to death. Knott administered oxygen intravenously to all of them. The results showed 50 percent of the comatose patients—those who were near death—recovered, and nearly 100 percent of the moderately ill people recovered.

Oxygen therapy has been used successfully to treat patients with staph infections, pneumonia, polio, and tuberculosis. Recently, it has shown good results in curing MRSA—the disease that people get in hospitals for which there is no known cure. A review of hundreds of cases of serious infections cured by oxygen therapy in the 1940s showed that it was effective, and had long-lasting results with no adverse effects. Which of our modern treatments can claim that?

Today, oxygen therapists use ozone therapy, hydrogen peroxide therapy (which utilizes a reactive form of oxygen [03]), and hyperbaric oxygen therapy. Increasing oxygenation is a powerful stimulant for healing, and it has anti-bacterial and anti-viral properties. Dr. Robert Rowen and others feel that this therapy can be very helpful in treating macular degeneration, glaucoma, and other eye disorders. Typically, twenty to forty treatments are necessary, although patients can experience benefits after just a few treatments. There are three major oxygen-related therapies:

- Ozone therapy (patients' blood is withdrawn, altered, and re-injected)
- Hydrogen peroxide therapy (patients are put on intravenous drips)
- Hyperbaric oxygen chambers (patients breathe pressurized, pure oxygen)

In the following sections, I discuss each therapy in more detail.

Ozone Therapy

What is ozone, precisely? If you've ever noticed the clean smell in the air after a lightning storm, then you know what ozone smells like; you were smelling ozone gas that had reacted with the atmosphere. This gas has a purifying and stimulating effect on people. The oxygen molecule is composed of two oxygen atoms. When an oxygen molecule is charged and acquires more energy, it attracts another oxygen atom and forms a three-molecule structure: ozone. So, ozone is similar to supercharged oxygen.

Ozone therapy is in the therapy class called oxidative therapy. In this therapy, the charged ozone molecules act as a catalyst to stimulate healing. If oxygen is good, ozone is much better! Studies show ozone therapy is very effective in treating both bacterial and viral infections. I believe, for example, that is one of the most effective and safe ways to treat flu symptoms. The last time I developed flu symptoms, all my symptoms disappeared after I had two oxidative treatments. The treatments stopped the virus cold in its tracks

Professor Velio Bocci, author of the textbook *Ozone Therapy* states that ozone therapy is based on exposing patients' blood to precise ozone concentrations. While some 95 to 98 percent of oxygen is always present, the real drug remains ozone, a highly reactive form of oxygen. Over the last ten years, Dr. Bocci's research has established a comprehensive framework for understanding ozone therapy use when treating select diseases.

Ozone therapy involves the introduction of ozone into the bloodstream. The therapist withdraws a small amount of blood from the patient, mixes it with ozone, and returns it to the patient. This activates the white blood cells, so they can kill any pathogens. Since the pathogens in the blood are killed when the ozone is administered, this therapy may also work by stimulating the immune system to recognize killed pathogens, acting as kind of auto-vaccine.

Hydrogen Peroxide Therapy

Hydrogen peroxide therapy is given to patients directly into the bloodstream, through a slow IV drip, and has the same good results as ozone therapy.

Hyperbaric Oxygen Therapy

Hyperbaric oxygen therapy (HBOT) uses a pressurized chamber to deliver oxygen under pressure to individuals who are lying within it. The patient is surrounded by and breathes in 100 percent pure oxygen. The typical treatment lasts for one hour. The patient is conscious at all times, but may sleep if he or she wishes. A typical course of treatment is ten treatments, and the effects can be noticed for up to one year.

Research proves that patients with many types of conditions respond well to this therapy; however, its use in conventional medicine is restricted to a few situations, such as treating divers who have "the bends" and some head injury and stroke victims.

Yet this treatment has been proven effective for a number of different medical and surgical conditions, either as a primary or adjunctive treatment. It is also used to treat many other medical conditions, even though it is a treatment that the mainstream still considers experimental. On his website, Dr. Elmer Cranton maintains a list of the many conditions that have been affected by this therapy. Most of them are life threatening and many do not have any known, effective, conventional treatment.

It is unlikely that your (conventional) doctor will prescribe this treatment and very unlikely that your insurance company will pay for it. Dr. Cranton makes this observation about HBOT:

Some day, when HBOT . . . is an established part of standard medical care, historians of twentieth-century medicine will wonder how so much supportive research on its benefits could have been published by skillful medical researchers and even more scrupulously ignored by the guardians of our health. By that time, most of the individuals who attempted to keep HBOT on the fringe will probably not be alive to blush, sparing them extensive embarrassment. (www.drcranton.com)

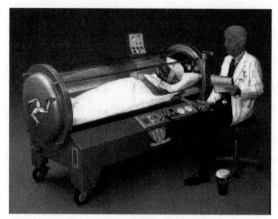

Hyperbaric oxygen chamber with patient and attendant.

Following is a list of eye conditions that Dr. Cranton says patients can improve with HBOT:

- Diabetic retinopathy
- Glaucoma with visual field loss
- Retinal artery occlusion
- Retinal vein thrombosis

I would add that HBOT slows the progression of macular degeneration.

As previously mentioned, it can be difficult to find a practitioner who will administer oxygen therapies to you. Some of my patients, who wish to self-administer this therapy, have purchased specialized equipment from my office. I urge anyone with a serious chronic condition or infection to investigate these methods of healing. In addition to the resolution of their infections and/or inflammation, people who receive oxygen treatments show lowering of blood pressure, improved cholesterol metabolism, improved kidney function, and better oxygen delivery to cells and tissues.

Recently, I treated a macular degeneration patient who is from Colorado and lives at 5,000 feet. I have another macular degeneration patient who is from Arizona's White Mountains and lives at 6,500 feet. When comparing these two patients, several questions came into my mind. What are the effects of low oxygen saturations at these altitudes? Does this contribute to the development of macular degeneration? What are the effects at high altitude? Oxygen saturation is reduced by 20 percent at 5,000 feet and by 30 percent at 10,000 feet. This reduction in oxygen saturation can be a problem for eye health, especially if the patient is subject to other conditions that affect oxygen use. Will increasing a patient's oxygen saturation help improve vision, then? Could hyperbaric oxygen treatment help patients' conditions at high altitudes?

Oxygen is essential to good health; low oxygen saturation in tissues will cause disease. Medical literature has clearly documented that people with low oxygen saturation will have greater occurrences of macular degeneration. Causes of low oxygen saturation include high altitudes, sleep apnea, tobacco abuse, and chronic pulmonary disease. All of these conditions will reduce the body's oxygen saturation.

Any condition that reduces the oxygen saturation needs to be corrected. At our practice, all of the patients being treated for macular degeneration and other eye problems are evaluated to determine any conditions that may be reducing their oxygen saturation. Low oxygen saturation is more common at night, especially in patients who have sleep apnea, lung disease, or chronic sinus infections. To measure the possible oxygen deprivation that may occur at night, we use a simple test, nocturnal pulse oximetry, which measures oxygen saturations. Finding a low value is a call to evaluate and treat the reason.

How can hyperbaric oxygen therapy correct low oxygen saturation? Placing someone in a pressured hyperbaric environment increases the atmospheric pressure, which increases the oxygen gas's partial pressure and thus forces the blood plasma to dissolve more oxygen. This saturation of oxygen in the blood allows extra oxygen to be diffused or transported to the surrounding body tissues. Thus, plasma transportation of oxygen significantly increases under hyperbaric therapy (HBOT). The following article, reprinted courtesy of Dr. Robert Rowen, summarizes HBOT research that all diabetics should find interesting. The article reveals oxygen therapy has good results in treating diabetes-induced damage to the eyes and kidneys.

Reverse Diabetic Retinopathy with Easy, In-Home Treatment

By Dr. Robert Rown, MD

You can reverse the two most-feared complications from diabetes, retinopathy, and nephropathy with a simple treatment you can do in your own home.

Both of these conditions [the complications] develop in diabetics because the disease causes the capillary membranes to thicken. When these membranes thicken, it hinders oxygen and nutrient delivery to the cells.

Unfortunately, conventional medicine has little to offer diabetics who develop these conditions. Most of them receive laser surgery, with little success. But a new study gives evidence that diabetics, even those who have had laser surgery, can benefit from one of my favorite therapies.

In a pilot study just published by Johns Hopkins Hospital, five patients between the ages of 52 and 69 with diabetic retinopathy were selected. All had conventional laser treatment previously and 9 of 10 eyes had persistent edema despite the laser. (Lasers burn abnormal and leaking blood vessels caused by diabetes in the retina.)

The patients were given supplemental oxygen (using an oxygen concentrator) at four liters per minute by nasal tube. They were instructed to use the oxygen continually for three months, except when taking showers.

At the end of the test period, extra thickness of the macula (your [area of] central vision) was reduced by 54 percent! Additionally, three of the eyes had better visual acuity, improving two lines on the reading chart. Most of the eyes gradually worsened when the oxygen was withdrawn. However, four of the eyes maintained stability, suggesting that supplemental oxygen has a stabilizing effect on the laser surgery for retinopathy.

The principal investigators in the study believe the retina, when faced with a decrease in oxygen, becomes leaky. This stimulates the growth of new (but abnormal) blood vessels.

Since the new blood vessels are abnormal, they can leak or bleed. So their presence is more dangerous to the eyes than simply needing the oxygen [is]. The leakage can cause the macula to become thickened, resulting in vision loss. This affects up to 10 percent of all patients with diabetes.

Supplemental oxygen prevents the eye from producing these abnormal vessels. This, in turn, reduces the amount of leaking in retinal vessels and prevents the macula from thickening. The treatment could reduce the thickness of the retina before laser treatment.

Burdened by less edema, laser treatment may become more effective, even when oxygen is withdrawn.

If you have diabetic retinopathy, or nephropathy, oxygen therapy is a must. In fact, if you have diabetes, you're most likely to have problems [to] some degree in many organs of the body. Don't wait for complications. Start EWOT today! And if you have diabetic complications, take this information to your doctor and ask to be prescribed supplemental oxygen. For more information on EWOT, please call 800-728-2288 and ask for my special report!

Reference:

Nguyen, Q.D., et al. "Supplemental Oxygen Improves Diabetic Macular Edema: A Pilot Study," *Investigative Ophthalmology & Visual Science* 45(2) (February 2004): 617-624.

The therapies described in this chapter aim to support cells and tissues at an essential level. Just as we discussed the importance of hydrating tissues, we are now discussing something even more elemental—oxygenating them. After all, there are reasons why specific diseases develop in specific people. It is not random. Of course, genetics can play a role in increasing the likelihood of a disease developing, but genetics do not predetermine situations. To a great extent, macular degeneration, glaucoma, and cataracts are problems caused by aging, poorly nourished, and poorly oxygenated tissues. Rarely do patients present with one of these diseases without having any of these other chronic conditions. Typically, patients with these eye problems are sedentary, eat the SAD (Standard American Diet), have used or currently use toxins in their environments, and test positively for heavy metal loads. We cannot simply intervene and "fix" an eye disease without changing the environment that produced it. That is why I have developed the holistic approach to treating eye disease described in this book.

I know that many, if not all, of the therapies described in this chapter may be new to you. However, that does not mean that these therapies have just been discovered. It means that mainstream doctors have still not accepted them. This does not mean that these therapies are not effective—far from it! If you want to restore your health and your vision, I suggest that you explore using at least one of these powerful methods to do so.

CHAPTER NINE NOTES

Ozone Therapy: Reports of Ozone Benefiting Macular Degeneration in European Studies

Sanseverino, Riva E., et al. "Effects of Oxygen-Ozone Therapy on Age-Related Degenerative Retinal Maculopathy." *Panminerva Medica* 32, no. 2 (Apr. – Jun. 1990): 77-84.

Summary: The results indicate that the majority of patients showed improvement in their ocular condition, which suggests the continuation of this type of investigation on a larger group of people.

In the United Kingdom, there are about 200,000 patients who have the atrophic dry form of macular degeneration; for these patients, ophthalmologists can only prescribe antioxidants and zinc, which do not harm but are ineffective. During the last eight years, researchers in Siena, Italy have treated hundreds of patients, achieving a significant improvement in about 70 percent of the cases. Usually patients who have fifteen treatments (one treatment twice weekly) and follow this treatment with maintenance therapy can retain sufficient vision acuity for many years.

Soto, G., et al. "Ozone Therapy in Senile Macular Degeneration."

Summary: Researchers performed a retrospective study on twenty-two patients who were assisted at the Ophthalmologic Service of the Medical Surgical Research Center (CIMEQ).

Centro de Investigaciones Médico Quirúrgicas, CUBA. The results demonstrated that of the patients treated with ozone, 80 percent had improvement of their visual acuity (with an average of 20% improvement in visual). Ozone therapy could be a good therapeutic choice for patients suffering from dry-type of macular degeneration.

Author's note: Although no formal studies have yet examined ozone's effects in treating glaucoma, I have observed that ozone therapy can stimulate the optic nerve's function, thereby stimulating healing and improving vision.

Several well-known alternative doctors, including Robert Rowen, M.D., and Frank Shallenberger, M.D., believe ozone therapy should be considered as a front-line attack in helping patients with macular degeneration. Typically, my colleagues and I will do two oxidative treatments during our three-day eye care program, but most authorities suggest between twenty and forty treatments for maximum effect. The problem is the cost; at $100 a treatment, this can be expensive.

Hyperbaric Oxygen Therapy

Robert Rowen, M.D., mentions a report by Drs. Jansen and Nielson (from Copenhagen, Denmark), which details two case histories of ARMD patients improving with hyperbaric oxygen treatment (HBOT). Both patients had cystoid macular degeneration. One patient, a Type-2 diabetic, went from a degree of visual acuity of 0.5 (he had difficulty reading) to 1.0 (he could read normally) with just one treatment. The second patient's visual acuity was only

0.2; he could not read at all. After five sessions of HBOT in three days, his acuity reached 0.9 and he could read normally. These doctors saw a "very rapid," day-by-day improvement in the patients' maculae; they recommend that treatment be started as early as possible, before there is irreversible damage.

Bojic, L., et al. "Hyperbaric Oxygenation in the Treatment of Macular Degeneration." Split, Yugoslavia: Split Naval Medical Institute, pp. 1-4. Selected References to Published Research on HBOT at http://drcranton. com/hbo/hbobib.htm.

Summary: In a clinical trial, four patients with advanced macular degeneration and severe vision loss received HBOT treatment. Three of the four patients experienced a doubling of visual acuity after HBOT.

Halit, Oguz, and Sobaci Gungor. "The Use of Hyperbaric Oxygen Therapy in Ophthalmology." *Survey of Ophthalmology* 53, no. 2 (Mar. - Apr. 2008): 112-20.

Abstract: Hyperbaric oxygen therapy is a primary or secondary adjuvant therapeutic method used in treatment of various acute or chronic disorders. Currently, eye diseases are among those receiving the off-label use of hyperbaric oxygen. However, there is increasing evidence showing hyperbaric oxygen treatment's safety and efficacy for the treatment of blocked arteries of the eye, swelling of the retina and non-healing ulcers of the eye. Recent studies point out its potential to treat some blinding diseases. This article constitutes an up-to-date summary of knowledge about the therapeutic use of hyperbaric oxygen, and aims to contribute further understanding of this therapy's current and potential use in ophthalmology.

Jansen, E.C., and N.V. Nielsen. "Promising Visual Improvement of Cystoid Macular Oedema by Hyperbaric Oxygen Therapy." *Acta Ophthalmologica Scandinavia* 82, no. 4 (Aug. 2004): 485-6.

Kurok, A.M., Kitaoka, T., Taniguchi, H., and T. Amemiya. "Hyperbaric Oxygen Therapy Reduces Visual Field Defect After Macular Hole Surgery." *Ophthalmic Surgery, Lasers & Imaging* (May - Jun. 2002): 200-6.

Weiss, J.N. "Hyperbaric Oxygen Therapy and Age-Related Macular Degeneration." *Undersea and Hyperbaric Medicine Journal* 37, no. 5 (Sep. - Oct. 2010: 375.
Abstract: Age-related macular degeneration (AMD) is a significant cause of visual loss in the United States and Western Europe. As the population ages, researchers expect the prevalence rate of advanced AMD by 2030. In this study, researchers used a one-hour session of hyperbaric oxygen therapy (HBO2) to treat a group of fourteen patients who had advanced AMD. Researchers observed significant improvements in visual acuity and/or visual fields, along with improvements in the activities of daily living.

EWOT: Exercise with Oxygen

Author's note: Obviously, your most important nutrient is oxygen! Exercise with oxygen therapy (EWOT), which has been performed for decades in Germany, is the granddaddy of oxygen therapies, and more proof of oxygen's value. Aging causes thickening of the capillaries. Years ago, researchers showed supplemental oxygen could reduce edema accumulated in the capillary-lining cells. This research confirms EWOT's power, but it may be decades before "modern" medicine accepts it.

How to Do EWOT (summarized from www.EWOT.com)

Purchase an oxygen generator (no prescription needed), which is a small portable device that plugs into the wall and produces 94-95 percent pure oxygen. (This does not require oxygen tanks, but uses your room air, removing the nitrogen and producing high oxygen purity.) A seven-foot tube connects to the machine and then goes over the ears and under the nose to supply oxygen. A person who wears the tube while exercising (e.g. riding an exercise bike or using an elliptical or whole-body vibration trainer [such as a TurboSonic, similar to the Power Plate described in Chapter Four]) will breathe approximately 20 percent higher levels of oxygen. With an oxygen mask the person can almost double the oxygen intake to between 35-40 percent. EWOT increases strength during the same time period, allowing the person to perform at a higher level and burn more calories. EWOT can make the difference between aging faster and slowing aging to a crawl. Practitioners suggest doing EWOT for fifteen minutes, three times a week—or more, if possible.

Websites

American College of Alternative Medicine

www.acam.org

CHAPTER 10

Stem Cell Therapy to Treat Eye Disease

Recently, both patients and practitioners have become interested in using stem cell therapy to treat macular degeneration and other health problems. A great deal of misinformation and controversy exists regarding stem cells and the sources for obtaining these cells. My interest in the subject originates from a conversation I had with Dr. Robert Rowen, who shared his father's positive experience with having stem cell therapy treatment for macular degeneration. This led me to visit the oldest stem cell center in Europe, the XCell-Center, which is in Düsseldorf, Germany. The country has very strict requirements about using stem cells. Even though they are processed from an individual's bone marrow, stem cells are considered a drug and must meet all the country's standards for drug approval.

To treat neurological conditions by using stem cells, a patient's cells must be harvested through bone marrow aspiration. Typically, the practitioner will take cells from the large hipbone. Then, using a proprietary process at a specialized lab, the cells are processed and become concentrated. In most neurological cases, the practitioner injects the stem cells directly into the patient's lumbar spinal canal. Dr. Cornelis Kleinbloesem, who is the medical director of the center, feels that this administration route will transmit the stem cells directly into the spinal fluid, which bathes the neurological tissues.

The center I visited currently averages around ten eye cases a week. The preferred method of administering stem cells, according the to the center's eye surgeon, Dr. Sassmanhausen, is retrobulbar injection. This type of injection does not go directly into the eye; instead, the injection goes under the eye and places the stem cells adjacent to the macular area. The XCell-Center plans to begin doing intraocular injections of stem cells, much like the method of injecting Avastin and Lucentis to treat wet macular degeneration. According to this method, the stem cells will be much closer to the retina, which will increase their beneficial effect.

The XCell-Center has treated over 200 cases of macular degeneration by using stem cells, and the statistics can be summed up as follows: one-third of the patients do fantastically well, one-third have a good response, and one-third have no response. During my visit, Dr. Kleinbloesem and I discussed alternative methods, like microcurrent, to help improve the stem cell therapy's results.

Shortly after my visit to the XCell-Center, I also spoke with David Steenblock, M.D., the author of *Umbilical Cord Stem Cell Therapy*. My research has led me to the conclusion that stem cells certainly can be beneficial in treating macular degeneration, and that microcurrent stimulation can be an important ancillary tool in insuring the success of the stem cell transplantation. Dr. Steenblock has made great advancements in the treatment of macular degeneration, glaucoma, and other eye diseases through stem cell therapy, and I am working with him to help advance this new type of therapy. Through the research and efforts of leaders in stem cell research, it is not necessary for patients to travel to Europe in order to take advantage of the most advanced techniques.

My close friend Gabriel Howearth (a botanist, landscape architect, and seedsman) tragically endured a debilitating stroke after suffering a long series of complications from a fungal infection. Gabriel used to be the owner of Seeds of Change, a company dedicated to preserving the world's seed lineage. He introduced me to the importance of organic gardening and natural herbal medicines. The stroke caused paralysis on one side of his body, which severely affected his ability to continue his brilliant work. Microcurrent therapy had helped him to some degree, but stem cell therapy was his last option.

Gabriel underwent stem cell therapy in 2011, under the direction of Dr. Steenblock, and his recovery has been remarkable. He is now back working in his garden, "Buena

Fortuna," in La Ribera, Mexico. He recently sent me a picture of himself in his garden, lifting a large log over his head.

WHAT ARE STEM CELLS?

With so much controversy and general misunderstanding surrounding stem cell therapy, I feel an obligation to offer you some basic information about it. First, it is important to understand what stem cells are. Stem cells are undifferentiated cells that have the potential to help repair and replace tissues anywhere in the body. These cells also have the potential to grow into specific body parts. Stem cells can initially be differentiated into three types of cells: ectoderm (skin, neurological tissue, and the eye), mesoderm (muscles, bones, and heart), and endoderm (lining of the gut and internal organs). After that initial differentiation, these types of cells then further develop into specific types of tissue.

Next, it helps to understand how stem cells work. Stem cells are constantly at work helping the body repair itself after injury, stress, and disease. One way this stem cell repair takes place is when hypoxic tissues (tissues with low oxygen and inflammation) attract stem cells. The stem cells begin replicating the specific cells in that area and aid the damaged tissue in repairing itself. For example, when you sustain a cut, stem cells can play a role in helping the cut tissue to regenerate. A salamander that has had a limb amputated is also a good example. Because of stem cells, the salamander has the ability to regenerate its limb.

In order for stem cells to work, they must be in undifferentiated states, so that they can evolve into the specific tissue(s) needed. Once stem cells develop into a specific tissue, they cannot go backwards or return to their previous states. This is a reason why doctors use undifferentiated stem cells in treatment; these cells have the greatest regenerative potential.

Types of Stem Cells

Medical practitioners around the world are currently using four main types of stem cells. The most common type of stem cell, and the first to be used, is called an *Allogenic Stem Cell*. ("*Allo*" means "other.") These are stem cells taken from one individual's (the donor's) bone marrow and then transplanted into another person (the recipient). Practitioners first used this type of transplantation in the treatment of leukemia. The tissues of the donor and recipient must be carefully matched in order to help prevent rejection.

The second type of stem cell is an *Autogenic Stem Cell*. ("*Auto*" means "self.") These stem cells are taken from the patient's own body (commonly from bone marrow, blood, or fat cells). These stem cells are treated, processed, and then injected back into the same patient. The medical goal here is that these concentrated stem cells will work on repairing diseased or damaged tissue.

The third type is a *Human Cord Stem Cell* (HCSC). These stem cells are taken from an umbilical cord immediately after a child's birth. These cells are extremely active and have a very low chance of rejection. Unfortunately, the FDA has only approved them for treating cases of leukemia and other blood disorders. In clinics overseas and in Mexico, patients are receiving HCSC as treatment for additional disorders. Dr. Steenblock and other specialists in this field believe that when a patient's autogenic stem cells are of poor quality, the patient should consider the option of using HCSC.

The fourth type of stem cell, and the most controversial, is an *Embryonic Stem Cell.* These are cells removed from an aborted fetus, and their use is currently outlawed in the United States and most other countries.

STEM CELLS AND EYE DISEASE

Dr. Steenblock has treated fifty macular degeneration patients with stem cells, using both autogenic stem cells (from the same patient) and human cord stem cells (from a newborn's umbilical cord). The majority of patients have had a marked improvement of vision. However, when evaluating this improvement in this series of patients, Dr. Steenblock did not measure visual parameters (acuity, contrast, visual fields and ocular tomography). To measure the benefits of stem cell therapy further, Dr. Steenblock and I will be collaborating on a study that carefully monitors visual parameters.

Stem Cells Regenerate a Mouse Retina

At the University of Washington, scientists have used human embryonic stem cells (from a line of cells approved in the United States) in a lab and added growth factors. The growth factors they added included proteins that enable cell growth, specifically cell growth that is central to the development of both human and mouse heads, as well as a growth factor essential to a frog's ability to sprout large eyes.

Within two weeks' time—that is, twice as fast as human cell development—the embryonic cells became "progenitor" (that is, forerunner) cells for retinal cells. The scientists injected these new cells into a damaged mouse retina, where the progenitor cells developed into cones (the retinal cells responsible for color), rods (the cells that allow night vision), and other cells. This research is ongoing. The scientists' next step will be to measure the nerve reactions within the repaired mouse retinas to see if the vision has improved.

Stem Cells and the Treatment of Corneal Disease

If the cornea's limbus area (the part where the cornea meets the sclera [white] of the eye) is injured or damaged, the number of proliferating stem cells can be reduced. Then, if the corneal stem cells are reduced or eliminated, the cornea experiences a gradual loss of transparency and scar tissue formation. Cord stem cell treatments may be beneficial for patients with this condition.

Stem Cells and the Treatment of Macular Disease

Recently, a practitioner used catheter surgery to place umbilical cord stem cells directly into the blood vessels that feed the macular area of a patient's eye. A week later, the person was able to see up-close images again after being blind for several years.

However, in cases where neovascularization (the formation of new blood vessels) is a part of the pathology, such as in patients who have wet macular degeneration and diabetic retinopathy, hyperbaric oxygen treatments may produce better results than stem cells. Generally, the initial cause of new blood vessel growth is a lack of oxygen. Oxygen and antioxidant treatments may help repair eye tissue without increasing the type of neovascularization that can interfere with the retinal center's visual field.

HOW IS STEM CELL THERAPY PERFORMED ON PATIENTS WITH MACULAR DEGENERATION?

Practitioners have developed three methods to administer stem cells in patients who have macular degeneration and other eye diseases. The most commonly used method is intravenous administration. Stem cells are injected into the blood stream through a catheter in the patient's arm. Dr. Steenblock prefers this method, and he has used it to treat many patients with macular degeneration. Most commonly, autogenic stem cells or human cord stem cells are used in this method.

The second method commonly used for administering stem cell therapy is retrobulbar injection (described above). A retrobulbar injection is a very common type of injection used in ophthalmology; it is delivered in the area under the eye (not in the eye), near the area of the macula. Finally, the third method now being used to administer stem cell therapy for the treatment of macular degeneration is an intraocular injection, or an injection placed directly into the eye. This is the method retinal doctors currently use to inject Avastin or Lucentis into patients' eye to treat wet macular degeneration. The benefit of this form of treatment is a higher concentration of stems cells near the macula. This method connects to a technique being further developed by Pfizer Pharmaceutical Company, which is working on a stem cell membrane that can be surgically implanted on the area of the macula. This type of implantation will be the fourth method of treatment.

Stem Cells and Retinal Disorders

Diseases that affect the outer retina usually cause retinal pigment epithelium (RPE) dysfunction. If an eye care practitioner can replace the damaged part with neuro-blastic progenitors, he or she may be able to prevent vision loss. In different animal models of retinal degeneration, retinal transplants can reconstruct damaged retinas and restore visual sensitivity. A retinal transplantation involves the rescue of host cones and the establishment of synaptic connectivity between the transplant and the host retina.

Microcurrent Improves Stem Cell Therapy's Effects

We have good, strong evidence that microcurrent treatment will improve stem cell function after transplantation. Numerous published research articles support this finding, showing that microcurrent improves circulation and stimulates cellular activity. Microcurrent stimulation alone promotes rapid results of stem therapy in macular degeneration patients. As I have written here and in previous books, microcurrent stimulation alone is a very valuable aid for reducing and reversing macular degeneration's effects. In the case of a patient who has undergone stem cell transplantation, microcurrent can increase cellular activity around the eye, thereby bringing blood and nutrients to the area and enhancing the stem cell's healing response. Microcurrent is a wonderful adjunctive therapy to employ after stem cells have been transplanted and the healing has begun.

PROPER PREPARATION IS KEY TO SUCCESS IN STEM CELL THERAPY

There are several keys to successful stem cell therapy. When a farmer plants seeds in a field, certain conditions must exist for those seeds to grow and thrive. Similarly, stem cells need a specific environment in which they can regenerate. Many of these keys to success are the same ones that I have observed improve the results of microcurrent therapy, and which I have discussed throughout this book.

First, a proper diet is essential! I recommend maintaining an all-organic (largely raw) diet that eliminates genetically modified organisms (GMO foods), gluten, dairy, coffee, and alcoholic beverages. This is especially important during the first several weeks after initiation of stem cell therapy.

Next, patients need to reduce the toxic load in their bodies. Before undergoing stem cell therapy, you must eliminate any heavy metals in your body. Heavy metals may interfere with the stem cells' replication and therefore hamper the therapy's success. It is routine for all patients to take a six-hour, heavy metal urine challenge test and then undergo chelation therapy, if needed, before their stem cell transplant procedures.

The next condition is adequate oxygenation. Proper oxygenation is essential for cell growth. Each person who wishes to be a candidate for stem cell therapy must have his or her oxygen saturation measured. Dr. Steenblock and I perform a nocturnal oxymetry text. This test measures oxygen saturation at night while the patient is asleep. We have found that many patients have low levels of oxygen at night because of obstructive airway disease (sleep apnea); this can contribute to eye disease development and, if not treated, can affect the success of other treatments. If a patient's oxygen saturation is low, he or she will likely need supplemental oxygen.

Lastly, all chronic infections, held anywhere in the body, must be eliminated. Stem cells tend to migrate to areas of inflammation and infection. Dr. Steenblock has observed that 50 percent of macular degeneration patients who do not respond well to stem cell therapy suffer from undiagnosed chronic sinus infections. Therefore, all patients with macular degeneration who are interested in undergoing stem cell therapy must first undergo either thermography (testing that identifies areas of inflammation without using of radiation) or a CT scan of the sinuses to rule out infection.

STEM CELL THERAPY: WHAT TO EXPECT NEXT

As you can see, at the time of this book's preparation, stem cell therapy for the treatment of eye disease is evolving very quickly. Not surprisingly, the United States lags behind other countries in stem cell research, so we need to stay informed of developments outside our borders. I believe that as baby boomers age and start developing degenerative eye conditions (including macular degeneration), we will find many more suitable candidates for this therapy in patients who have, aside from their eye conditions, good health overall. As research in other promising areas of stem cell use develops—such as the use of stem cells to treat spinal cord injuries and heart disease—the applications of stem cell use in eye disease treatment will accelerate.

About the Author

Dr. Kondrot is the world's leading homeopathic ophthalmologist. He devotes his practice to traditional and alternative therapies for treating eye disease. His extensive research has taken him around the world and placed him in a unique position to share this knowledge. Dr. Kondrot's two best selling books, *Healing the Eye the Natural Way* and *Microcurrent Stimulation: Miracle Eye Cure*, share this knowledge. Both books are solid introductions to his philosophy and practice. He also hosts Healthy Vision Talk Radio, a weekly radio show educating people about alternative treatments for eye disease.

Dr. Kondrot's prestigious eye care center, Healing the Eye, promotes wellness of sight, body, mind, and spirit, and is located near Tampa, Florida. The center treats patients who seek holistic, non-invasive therapies for eye problems that include macular degeneration, glaucoma, cataracts, eyestrain, and other eye disorders. Dr. Kondrot has a worldwide following because of these successful therapies.

Dr. Kondrot's achievements include:

- practicing ophthalmology for over twenty years and classical homeopathy for over fifteen years
- receiving his M.D. in 1977 from Hahnemann Medical College in Philadelphia, Pennsylvania
- completing his residency in ophthalmology at the Scheie Eye Institute in Philadelphia, Pennsylvania, and at St. Francis General Hospital

in Pittsburgh, Pennsylvania, becoming a board-certified ophthalmologist in 1981

- receiving his diploma from the Hahnemann Homeopathic College in Albany, California, in 1995
- becoming certified by the Council of Homeopathic Certification in 2000
- becoming a Doctor of Homeopathic Therapeutics (DHt) in 2002
- holding active medical licenses in Arizona, California, Florida, and Pennsylvania

Dr. Kondrot can be reached at:
1 (800) 430-9328
drkondrot@healingtheeye.com
www.healingtheeye.com

Dr. Kondrot's Exclusive Program to Improve Your Eyesight

The Kondrot Program Includes the Following:

- Limo Service from the Tampa Airport
- Boot Camp to Restore your vision
- 3 day accommodations and all healthy organic meals at the Florida Wellness Center
- Comprehensive eye exam and testing
- Homeopathic evaluation
- 3 days of treatment (4 microcurrent treatments and 2 light treatments daily)
- Personalized microcurrent machine with 5 programs
- Light therapy equipment
- Rectal ozone insuflation equipment.
- One month and 3 month telephone follow ups
- 6 month return visit to the Center which includes limo service form the airport, 2 days accommodations and healthy organic meals at the center.
- One year of reprogramming of microcurrent machine
- Light therapy glasses
- One year supply of ocular vitamins, homeopathic remedy and detox vitamins
- Instructional material including educational DVD
- telephone support

The cost includes all of ancillary treatments such as hyperbaric oxygen, Myers cocktail, ozone therapy and additional testing that might be needed at the center

Please call office for cost of the Kondrot Program.

Boot Camp Guarantee!

If you do not have an improvement in your vision after the 3 day boot camp program you will not be obligated to purchase the microcurrent machine and continue the program. It is our goal to help you improve your vision and quality of life.

Call for more information:
800-430-9328
info@HealingTheEye.com

Fast Track to Begin Microcurrent

With this program, you have no need to travel to another city.

The Fast Track to Begin Microcurrent program system includes:

1. A thorough review of your case history and eye records

2. A nutritional evaluation, including a zinc test and a six-hour urine test for heavy metals

3. DVD/CD Modules for Home Training, including:
   □ Nutrition and Vitamins for Your Eye Disease
   □ Hydration and Detox

Dear Reader,

Eyesight is a precious gift. When it's lost, you feel like you've lost a lot more than just your vision. I have created a special, free webinar that will help you through answering ten essential questions, including:

- What simple, practical things can I do on a daily basis to help my eyesight?
- What foods should I be eating and avoiding?
- What are the facts regarding stem cell therapy?
- What is homeopathy and how can it help my eye problem?
- Is there scientific evidence that microcurrent can improve vision?
- What is syntonic light therapy and how is it being used to stimulate stem cells?
- What are the best ways to detox the body?

You can register for this free webinar, "Ten Essentials to Save Your Sight," at http://www.healingtheeye.com/Webinar.html.

I have also created several other content-packed resources to help guide you in your journey to regaining your eyesight. You can find these (including "Pass Your Driver's Test!") on my website. I am continually adding content and new resources to my website, so I encourage you to visit it to find out about these.

Get your free resources at
http://www.healingtheeye.com/Webinar.html

You can also sign up for my newsletter, and receive many of these updates sent conveniently right to your inbox, here http://www.healingtheeye.com/newsletters.html

Are you looking for vitamins? It can be tough finding quality vitamins that truly help your health. I have created a list of recommended vitamins at http://www.healingtheeye.com/Vitamins.html

If you are looking for treatment programs, we offer two:
1. The 3-day in Office program. Get the details at http://www.healingtheeye.com/3day.html
2. The Fast Track Program to Begin Microcurrent (and other alternative methods to improve your vision). The Fast Track Program is home-based, so travel is not necessary. Get the details at http://www.healingtheeye.com/3day_Fast_Track.html

Here is what people have said after completing our 3-day in Office program:

"I like all of you! Dr. Kondrot is brilliant. I am able to see better in bright light and do not have to squint. I can see more color and it is easier to see without my glasses.

My vision improvement in three days was four letters [on the eye chart] in my right eye and eleven letters in the left eye."

-E.C. (patient with PVD and
diabetic retinopathy), Arizona

"I'm impressed with how much the staff cares and believes in what they are doing. The 'fog' has lifted. My vision improvement is seventeen letters in the right eye and five letters in the left eye."

-P.M. (patient with optic atrophy), Arizona

"I liked everything about this program. It gave me hope. My vision improvement is seven letters better in the right eye and eight letters better in the left."

-J.D. (patient with ARMD), Arizona

You can find more information on my website:
www.healingtheeye.com
or call my office for more details:
1 (800) 430-9328

To your good health and clear vision!
EDWARD C KONDROT, MD, MD(H), CCH, DHt
drkondrot@healingtheeye.com

P.S. Join me every Sunday evening for Healthy Vision Talk Radio. You can listen online and ask questions of our exciting array of guests. Listen in at http://www.healingtheeye.com/KFNX.html

P.P.S. Don't forget that you can get answers to ten essential questions about saving your sight in my free webinar at http://www.healingtheeye.com/Webinar.html

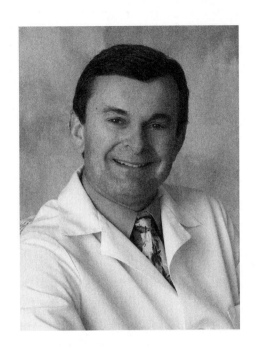

Dr. Kondrot is a sought after speaker and is available
for speaking engagements.

www.healingtheeye.com
1 (800) 430-9328

Index

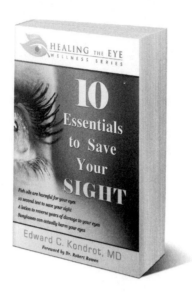

How can you use this book?

MOTIVATE

EDUCATE

THANK

INSPIRE

PROMOTE

CONNECT

Why have a custom version of *Ten Essentials to Save Your Sight?*

- Build personal bonds with customers, prospects, employees, donors, and key constituencies

- Develop a long-lasting reminder of your event, milestone, or celebration

- Provide a keepsake that inspires change in behavior and change in lives

- Deliver the ultimate "thank you" gift that remains on coffee tables and bookshelves

- Generate the "wow" factor

Books are thoughtful gifts that provide a genuine sentiment that other promotional items cannot express. They promote employee discussions and interaction, reinforce an event's meaning or location, and they make a lasting impression. Use your book to say "Thank You" and show people that you care.